Self
Study
for
Professional
Competence

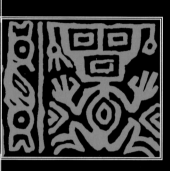

The

Health

Education

Specialist

Sigrid G. Deeds, Dr.P.H., C.H.E.S.

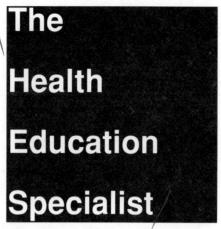

The Health Education Specialist

*Self Study
for Professional Competence*

SIGRID G. DEEDS, Dr.P.H., C.H.E.S.

The purpose of this outline is to guide your self study as you strengthen your skills in and knowledge of the processes of health education and add to your proficiency and professionalism. It is designed to assist your preparation to certify as an entry-level Health Education Specialist.

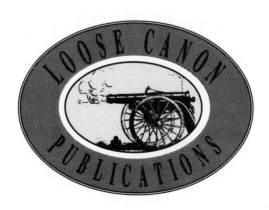

Written by Sigrid G. Deeds, Dr.P.H., C.H.E.S.

Published by Loose Canon Publications, P.O. Box 5538, Los Alamitos, Californi: 90721-5538. Telephone number (410) 430-2310. For further information or additional copies contact Dr. Deeds at the address above.

ISBN 1-881464-05-9

RA
440
.D43
1992

TABLE OF CONTENTS

"Remember always to be grateful for the millions of people everywhere whose despicable habits make health education necessary."

--- Mohan Singh

♦

THE HEALTH EDUCATION SPECIALIST
How to Improve Your Skills and Competence

This outline has been designed to assist the entry-level health educator qualify as a specialist in the areas of responsibility and competence that have been defined by the National Commission on Health Education Credentialing, Inc. The areas of responsibility provide the basic organization for the book. The wording of those statements taken from commission materials is written in italics.

The areas of responsibility for the entry-level Health Education Specialist are processes, rather than content in most cases. As you look at the wording of the National Commission on Health Education Credentialing, Inc.[1] documents, you see verbs such as advocate, decide, interpret, collaborate, develop, monitor, modify. In order to display competence in these activities , it is necessary to apply processes to specific examples. Therefore, in addition to reviewing the seven responsibilities/competencies, the major settings where Health Education Specialists are employed— community, school, medical care, and workplace–are given separate sections covering some special circumstances and issues that influence how you use these processes differently in one setting from another.

On your own, how do you improve your competence and judgment in an area? Read and discuss case studies, talk to practicing health educators about what they do and why they do it, read books, go to professional meetings. When you lead a discussion, plan a meeting, consult or give advice, don't be afraid to ask for feedback. The same is true of decision-making–ask why it's good or why it isn't!

Congratulations on taking a big step toward being a professional if you have decided to go for certification. Certification of Health Education Specialists provides peer recognition of quality performance which will advance our profession as it assures consumers of our services of the validity of our qualifications. More details on the areas of responsibility and the competencies can be found in A Framework for the Development of Competency-based Curricula for Entry Level Health Educators.[2] For information on this publication, the certification process, or the exam contact the Commission. The address is in Appendix III page 115.

Begin by rating yourself on the Self Assessment for Health Educators scale in the appendix to identify those areas in which you feel strong and weak. The exercise will help you organize your time and focus your learning opportunities. If your purpose in reviewing this outline is to prepare for the upcoming certification exam, you may wish to borrow or purchase textbooks now. Check the brief list of general references at the end of the outline. The examination focuses heavily on application and synthesis of the various areas of your training.

My advice is to read one or two books from start to finish so that you have a feel for the general organization and integration of basic health education concepts, rather than the details.

Then, if you have time, pursue specifics. Since one of the purposes of being a Health Educator is
organize communities and assess the health of populations, it's a good idea to include a book
introducing you to public health. And hearing about the exam questions, it appears to be a natura
in which to write items! Browsing through a couple of years of some of the major health educati
journals can give you a good feeling for perspective, evidence of effectiveness, and current issues
the trade. A list of journals that are important to our field is also included in the bibliography.

The selection of material, questions, and examples that follow does not represe
credentialing examination information from the Commission. It is based on two sources; one is r
judgment about appropriateness—y'know, if I were queen, this is what I'd include in the exam.
other source is exit interviews with examinees from the last two years. It is not the purpose of thi
manual to reprint all the information that is otherwise available to you but to identify and integrat
basic materials generally utilized in training professionals in health education. There are differen
of opinion, vocabulary, and definitions among authorities, as well as between school health,
community health, and medical care educators. Where possible, I have tried to flag some of the
concepts that can be interpreted several ways.

The test items, according to the NCHEC, are multiple choice. The examples
presented in this outline are a combination of questions that test takers remembered (probably be
they were the most difficult to answer) and items that I have created. With both types of items th
answer quite often should be "it depends." Unfortunately, that choice is not available, so you ha
use your best judgment. Keep in mind that "entry-level" assumes basic knowledge and skills, but
much experience.

The purpose of a number of my items is to provoke discussion rather than prov
rote answers. The exam changes every year. I am not providing my version of the answers beca
these items are intended to be used as the basis for study and discussion with your peers and your
instructors.

This outline attempts to provide breadth, rather than depth. The key is selectiv
what to include or exclude and how much detail to provide, while keeping this to a reasonable siz
strictly a judgment call. This is a work-in-progress. If you have suggestions for change, other cr
references, items that have been left out, I will appreciate hearing your comments. My address ca
found on the face page of the book.

SIGRID G. DEEDS

*Among the many who helped and encouraged me, I would like particularly to acknowledge
Ginger Hahn, Nancy Berkow Hassan, Inga Hoffman, Marion Pollock,
and my colleagues at CSU Long Beach.*

[1] National Commission for Health Education Credentialing, Inc.: Self Assessment for Health Educators, New York, 1987.
[2] A Framework for the Development of Competency-based Curricula for Entry Level Health Educators, 1985. Available through NCHEC

OUTLINE
The Context Of Health Education

1. What was the name of the famous Clair Turner study in the 1920's? a) the Malden Health Education study; b) Mortality Rates Among Italian-American Babies; c) Multiple Risk Factor Intervention Trials (MRFIT); d) the Framingham Study.

2. What is the least important factor in determining health status: a) medical care, b) heredity, c) environment, d) lifestyle behaviors.

3. According to the Surgeon General's Report, Healthy People..., which has the greatest potential for decreasing morbidity?
a) heredity, b) environment, c) lifestyle behaviors, d) available health care.

4. Healthy People: Year 2000 categorizes U.S. health issues according to:
a) primary, secondary, and tertiary prevention; b) health promotion, protection, and prevention; c) stages of development and health problems from infants to elderly; d) morbidity and disability in regions of the U.S.

5. Which of the following graphs reflects a measles epidemic?
a) b) c) d).

6. Which of the following graphs reflects endemic rabies in this community?
a) b) c) d).

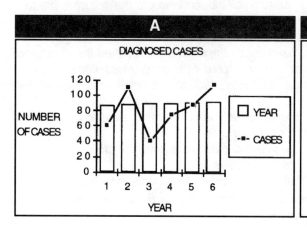

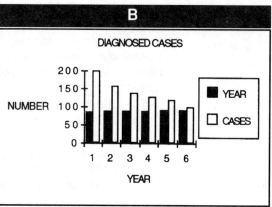

C	D

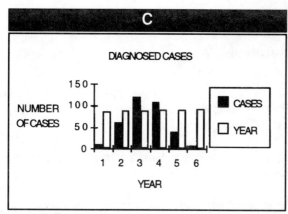

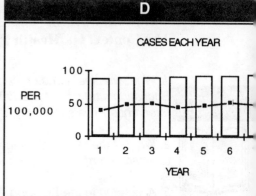

7. Review the graph on page 5 "Infectious and Chronic Disease Rates, U.S. 1900-1970" select the best response: a) chronic diseases have decreased in the population, b) acute diseases continue to kill a majority of the citizens, c) the U.S. is on the verge of eliminating the causes of mortality, comparing 1900 to 1970, d) death rates in this country have not changed much.

8. Two communities have the same crude death rate (8.7 per 1000). Select the correct statement from the following:
    a) Both communities will have similar age-adjusted death rates.
    b) Both communities will have approximately equal numbers of Latino deaths.
    c) If one community has more elderly people than the other it should have a higher crude death rate.
    d) Adding sex and age specific distributions would make it possible to study differences in the communities.

9. The phrase "excess deaths" expresses the difference between the number of deaths observed in a group and the number expected if the death rates were similar to the general population. Based on the last several years data select the incorrect statement from the following:
    a) Excess deaths for infant mortality among African Americans are four times higher than for Caucasians.
    b) Excess deaths for injury and accident are lower for males from 18-25 than they are for females.
    c) Excess deaths of Native Americans occur mostly after age 45.
    d) The major contributors to excess deaths for Black males are homicide and unintentional injury.

10. Rank unintentional injury among the leading causes of death in the U.S.

a) first, b) second, c) third, d) fourth.

11. Rank unintentional injury as a cause for age-specific mortality 1-35 years in the U.S.
a) first, b) second, c) third, d) fourth

12. Which of the following techniques is an example of secondary prevention?
a) health screening, b) immunization, c) chemotherapy, d) smoking cessation.

13. In the epidemiology of auto accidents, the driver's skills and knowledge are an example of: a) the host, b) the guest, c) the agent, d) the environment.

14. Which statistic is the.most sensitive reflection of a community's health?
a) HIV, b) unemployment, c) infant mortality, d) death rates.

15. You, the health education specialist, have been assigned to sit on the bioethics committee of an HMO. Select from the following, the responsibility that is not appropriate for your role: a) insure that informed consent statements are written at an appropriate level for the clientele; b) insure the confidentiality of medical examination data; c) recommend that reports developed are available to the population studied and to the public; d) screen interview instruments for cultural sensitivity.

16. The adult learner responds more to: a) traditional lectures, b) problem-solving, experiences, c) learning based on future developmental roles, d) reading assignments.

THE CONTEXT OF HEALTH EDUCATION

The last responsibility listed, Communication, (see Appendix II page 105) has three compete listed that set the context for the entire outline. Health education does not occur in a vacuur important for you to know the social, political, and economic context of our society both past an current that shaped our professional history and shapes our actions as well as our assumptions at health and disease. Therefore, I have put it at the beginning to give it the importance it deserves to set the stage for the processes.

N. C. H. E. S.
REQUIREMENT

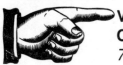

VII COMMUNICATE HEALTH AND HEALTH EDUCATION NEEDS, CONCERNS, AND RESOURCES

7.1 Keep abreast professional literature, current trends, and research
7.2 Advocate for inclusion of education in health programs and services
7.3 Explain the foundations of the discipline of health education including purposes, theories, history, ethics, and contributions in order to promote development and practice of health education.

A. HEALTH NEEDS AND CONCERNS

- HEALTH PRIORITIES IN 1992
    1. The ten major causes of death in the U.S. (See table 1 page 10)
    2. Year 2000: Objectives for the Nation (See page 117)
    3. Healthy Communities 2000: Model Standards *(1991)*
    4. The need for prevention. Focus has moved from 70's physician/medical care capacity building, 80's individual health promotion/wellness emphasis, to community/environmental resource allocation/quality of life issues related to prevention and promotion in 90's.
- FORCES SHAPING HEALTH TODAY
    1. Shift from acute to chronic diseases & theory of multicausality (See Figure 1 page 5)
    2. Costs
    3. Medical technology
    4. Demographics - population size, percentages, change- aging and immigration
    5. Telecommunications

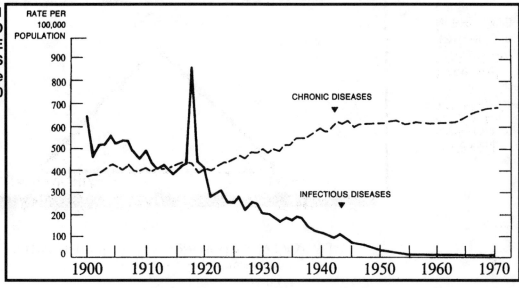

Figure 1
TIOUS AND
IC DISEASE
ATH RATES
in the
. 1900-1970

RATE PER
100,000
POPULATION

CHRONIC DISEASES

INFECTIOUS DISEASES

•TOOLS FOR COMMUNITY HEALTH STUDY
    1. Epidemiology - study of determinants and distribution of diseases in human populations (person, place, time). Determine causality & association.
    2. Demography–study of human populations - size, composition, distribution, density, growth, etc. and origins of change.
    (See page 11 for public health concepts)

Figure 2
LEVELS OF
REVENTION
diagram from
tt and Hanlon
(Pickett 1990)
shows the
relationship of
the levels of
vention to the
es of disease,
impairment,
disability and
dependency.

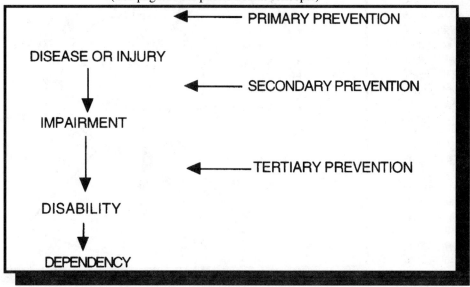

PRIMARY PREVENTION

DISEASE OR INJURY

SECONDARY PREVENTION

IMPAIRMENT

TERTIARY PREVENTION

DISABILITY

DEPENDENCY

**Figure 3
FACTORS IN
THE CONTROL
OF INFECTIOUS
DISEASES**
Infectious diseases
are controlled by
intervening at
one of these
three points

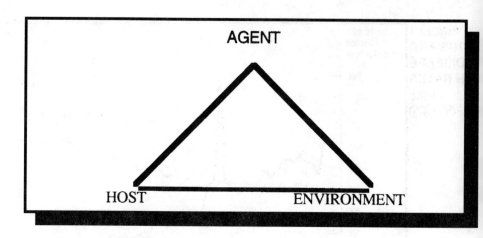

• FACTORS AFFECTING INDIVIDUAL HEALTH STATUS
1. Environment
2. Lifestyle
3. Biology–genetics, aging
4. Access to health care

**Figure 4
FACTORS
AFFECTING
INDIVIDUALS'
HEALTH**
Agencies and
individuals have
different views
about the amount
of influence each
of these factors
has on the health
of an individual
(ex. CDC attributes
over 50% of the
affect to lifestyle
whereas many
public health field
workers feel that
the social, cultural
& physical
environment rate the
largest share of the
attribution)

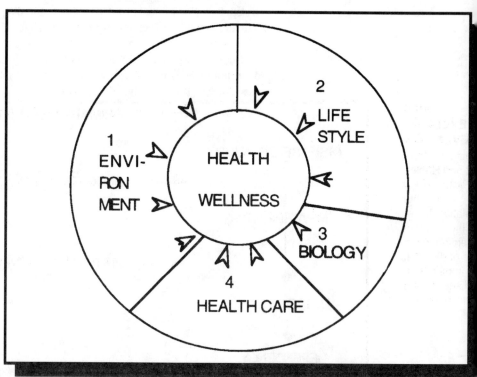

6

- DETERMINANTS OF INEQUITY IN HEALTH STATUS OF GROUPS
    1. Ethnicity
    2. Location
    3. Income
    4. Age
    5. Education
    6. Occupation

- THE PLAYERS IN THE HEALTH FIELD
    1. Major international agencies
    2. Federal government agencies
    3. Major voluntary agencies
    4. National health education associations

B. INTERPRET CONCEPTS, PURPOSES, THEORIES OF HEALTH EDUCATION PROCESS

- CHARACTERISTICS OF HEALTH EDUCATION
    1. Definitions (See page 9)
        a. Process
        b. Outcome
    2. Foundations of health education are education, biological, behavioral, sociological sciences and public health
    3. Learner/client oriented–philosophy & ethics
    4. Prevention and health promotion oriented
    5. Intangible - therefore, heavy emphasis on evaluation/accountability
    6. Scarce resources - therefore, focus on efficiency & effectiveness
    7. Professionalism

- PHILOSOPHY, PRINCIPLES, ETHICS OF HEALTH EDUCATION
    See page 15
- HISTORY
    See page 8

- THEORIES
    See Appendix I page 101

C. ADVOCATE FOR INCLUSION OF HEALTH EDUCATION

Community advocacy is a process used for social change. This process includ community organizing, coalition building, education of the community and the decision makers. Technical assistance and consultation may be used to build the capacity of community members groups to address health issues and influence social change.

Health education advocates recognize and address barriers that impede success health education interventions, promote self-help, community participation, capacity building, a health behavior change and show sensitivity to the needs of diverse populations.*(Standards of P 1991)*

Advocacy requires knowing a rationale for expenditure of resources Example: "The si most important contribution school health programs can make to promote health is to emphasize importance of lifestyles, and the environment, and to teach children how to use the health system Effective health education early in life can help to prevent the major diseases of adulthood. We learn even more about the development of living patterns at a young age, that will lead to healthi adult lives." *(Califano 1977)*

Advocacy for health education also requires knowing the successes in the field effectiveness of interventions and conditions required to achieve successful behavior change.

See page 20 for a list of studies that demonstrate effective health education.

§ HISTORY OF U.S. SCHOOL AND PUBLIC HEALTH EDUCATION §	1798... *U.S. Public Health Service begun as the Merchant Marines Hosp Service. Local health departments, Baltimore 1878, Charleston, 1815, Philadelphia 1818* 1837... *First of Horace Mann's Annual Reports campaigned for mandatory programs of hygiene*	1850-1900... *1850 Lemuel Shattu authored "Report of Sanitary Commission Massachusetts," aka "T Shattuck Report"* *1866 Stephen Smith, physician, and Dorma Eaton, a lawyer, wrote M Carta for health departn Their methods: gatheree urged backing of med profession, popular sup*

HEALTH EDUCATION DEFINITIONS

There are dozens of definitions of health education. The first one that follows was chosen because it was developed in the role delineation that grew into the current credentialing process.

> *1*
>
> *Health education is the process of assisting individuals, acting separately and collectively, to make informed decisions on matters affecting individual, family, and community health. Based upon scientific foundations, health education is a field of interest, a discipline, a profession.*
> *The Role Delineation Process*

The second one focuses on the important elements of the health education program process: designed (planned, not accidental) combination of methods (use more than one to be effective); voluntary (participants have choices) adaptations (we may wish to prevent, initiate, or sustain existing behavior not just change) of behavior.

> *2*
>
> *Health education is any designed combination of methods to facilitate voluntary adaptations of behavior conducive to health.*
> *Green et al., Health Education Planning*

and legislative action **1869 Massachusetts first true state Board of Health**	*Health departments focused on sanitation, control of epidemics, quarantine, fumigation, legal & policy issues*	**1901 Thomas D. Wood, M.D., "Father of health education" established program of professional preparation in hygiene at Columbia University**
Louis Pasteur (1857) discoveries from 1870-72	*Rapid growth of school health education, stimulated by Mann's writings, growth of voluntary agencies, child study movement, and pubic health*	*First of White House conferences on the health of children*
State Health Depts started: Louisiana Health Dept... 1855 - yellow fever epidemic Massachusetts 1869 Washington, D.C. 1870 Calif. & Virginia 1871	**1900's...** *Rise of health departments*	*1902 Public Health Service Act- organized Public Health*

Table 1
TEN LEADING
CAUSES OF
DEATH
IN THE
UNITED
STATES
National Center
for Health Statistics,
January 1991

Cause of Death	Percentage of total	Risk Factors
Heart Disease	38.1%	Smoking, hypertension, hypercholesterolemia, lack of ex◄ diabetes mellitus, obesity, stress
Cancer	21.9%	Smoking, alcohol, diet, environm carcinogens, obesity
Stroke	7.8%	Hypertension, smoking, hypercholesterolemia, stress
Accidents	4.5%	Alcohol, failure to use seat belts
Chronic obstructive lung disease	3.3%	Smoking
Pneumonia and influenza	2.7%	Smoking, alcohol
Diabetes mellitus	1.8%	Obesity
Suicide	1.4%	Stress, alcohol, drug use
Cirrhosis	1.4%	Alcohol
Atherosclerosis	1.3%	Smoking, hypercholesterolemia
Other	15%	
All causes	100%	

& Marine Hospital Service, renamed Public Health Service in 1912

1911 Creation of Joint Committee on Health Problems in Education (NEA & AMA)

1917 Involvement of the learner in the learning process

1918 American Child Health Assoc. established to improve the health of children

Voluntary health agencies (1918 National TB Assoc.; now American Lung Assoc.) Sally Lucas Jeans started health campaigns, Some efforts in public schools

New knowledge Kock, Lister discoveries

The Public Health Educators were writers, journalists, social workers, nurses (home visits)

focused on communic diseases, infant and ma mortality, poor sanit conditions. School health educar included in professio training programs in normal schools

Many babies died ◄ communicable diseases nutrition

1920's...

SCHOOL HEALTH EDUCATION CONCEPTS *(Pollock and Hamburg 1985)*

Health education is an applied science basic to the general education of all children and youth. Its body of knowledge represents a synthesis of facts, principles, and concepts drawn from biological, behavioral, sociological and health sciences, but interpreted in terms of human needs, human values, and human potential. Acquisition of information is a desired purpose but not the primary goal of instruction. Rather, growth in critical thinking ability and problem solving skills are both the process and the product of instruction...The ultimate goal of health education is the development of an adult whose lifestyle reflects actions that tend to promote his or her own health as well as that of family and the community.

School health starts from a developmental point of view of keeping healthy children healthy and giving them command of health knowledge and skills, using the individual or the classroom as the unit of analysis.

Public health on the other hand focuses on populations, the community and organizations. It starts from a health problem point of view, and assumes that the environment, social and political as well as physical, is a major aspect of ameliorating a problem.

PUBLIC HEALTH CONCEPTS

PREVENTION: Definition: anticipatory action taken to reduce the possibility of an event or condition occurring or developing, or to minimize the damage that may result from the event or condition if it does occur. *(Torjman: Prevention in the drug field. 1. Essential concepts and strategies. Toronto, Addiction Research Foundation, 1986)*

Primary prevention - Strategies to reduce the incidence of cases 1) make the host stronger and more resistant 2) decrease the effect of the agent upon the host 3) create a barrier in the environment.

1921 Mary Spencer, first student to complete all three degree programs in health education, was awarded Ph.D. by Columbia University

1921 MIT Health education training under Professor Claire Turner & W.T. Sedgwick M.D. at Harvard-MIT - started first MPH program; conducted Summerville and Malden Studies to clarify the status and

role of health education

1922 Public Health Education Section of APHA founded, Lecture, information giving, beginning use of advertising

1925 School health movement - school nurses hygiene education - physical examinations

Metropolitan Life Insurance Co. - Community Nurses to

help people take care of themselves.
Yale & N.C. Schools of Public Health introduced a course or major in health education

1930's...
1930 The beginning of the use of community organization; use of existing community groups - their resources and relationships (ex: PTA , voluntary agencies)

Secondary prevention - Objective to reduce prevalence Methods are screening and casefinding early detection, diagnosis and treatment to limit disability.

Tertiary prevention - Objective to slow progress of disease or avoid other complications of the process. Aim to reduce impact of existing conditions on the Quality of Life (QOL).
(Adapted from Pickett & Hanlon 1991)

See figures 2 & 3 pages 5 & 6.

EPIDEMIOLOGICAL TERMS:

Incidence = Number of new cases occurring during a defined time.

Prevalence = The number of cases in the community (state, world, etc.) at a given time.

Excess deaths expresses the difference between the number of deaths observed in a group and number expected if the death rates were similar to the general population.

Crude death rate is the total number of deaths at all ages in the jurisdiction for the year divided total number of people in the population at midpoint for that year (usually multiplied by 1000) Age specific death rates are defined as the deaths among residents (age X) in a specific year div by the population of the same age at midyear

    Example:

    deaths of children 1-5 in California in 1985

    —————————————————————— X 1000

      total # of children age 1-5 in CA. at midyear

1931 The Cattagaugus Study, directed by Ruth Grout, studied the impact of health education and the competency of health teachers

1935 Social Security Act passed

1936 The Astoria Study was directed by Dorothy Nyswander. All aspects of school health programs focusing on school health

services

1940's...

1940 Community organization demonstrations in North Carolina around war efforts and needs of workers (communicable diseases). Beginning of patient education Syphillis & gonorrhea - rapid treatment

1942-1963 Mayhew Derryberry, Chief of Health

Ed. Services (Ph.D. psychology), helped de training in behavioral and change

1943 School Comm. E Project in Michiga demonstrates effectiver comprehensive sche community health pro

1944 Similar progr demonstrated in Calif

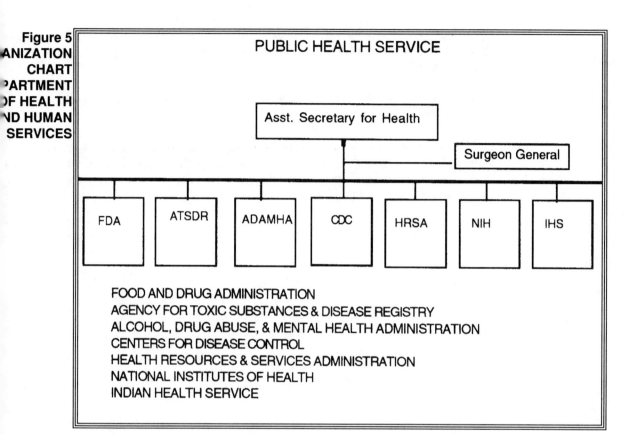

Figure 5
ORGANIZATION CHART DEPARTMENT OF HEALTH AND HUMAN SERVICES

PUBLIC HEALTH SERVICE

Asst. Secretary for Health

Surgeon General

FDA | ATSDR | ADAMHA | CDC | HRSA | NIH | IHS

FOOD AND DRUG ADMINISTRATION
AGENCY FOR TOXIC SUBSTANCES & DISEASE REGISTRY
ALCOHOL, DRUG ABUSE, & MENTAL HEALTH ADMINISTRATION
CENTERS FOR DISEASE CONTROL
HEALTH RESOURCES & SERVICES ADMINISTRATION
NATIONAL INSTITUTES OF HEALTH
INDIAN HEALTH SERVICE

1945 The Denver Interest Study, a needs assessment for the development of curriculum, was conducted

Definition of manpower for the Health Department local units
- Haven Emerson (Yale)
Ira Hiscock (Yale)
Beginnings of research efforts

Proliferation of health ed training programs in Schools of Public Health

1) UNC, Lucy Morgan (community organization)
2) Michigan, Mable Rugen (school)
3) Minnesota, Ruth Grout (school/comm)
4) UCB, Dorothy Nyswander (community & interpersonal processes)

Now had 25 accredited schools of public health

World War II ended officially

in 1946

1947 460 employed as health educators.
300 had completed graduate courses in recognized schools of public health. (This estimate does not include school health educators, colleges, PHNs, dentists, etc.)

1948 National Conference on Undergraduate Professional Preparation in Health, Phys

<u>*Screening:*</u> use of a test to separate a population group into two groups: one with higher than a chance of having or developing a specific disease or condition, and the other with a lower than average chance.

<u>*High risk group:*</u> Population with a higher than average chance of having or developing a spec disease or condition.

<u>*Risk factors:*</u> Characteristics or behavioral patterns that increase a person's risk of disease or disorders (particularly heart disease, stroke, cancer.) Risk factors can be divided into those tha be modified (age, sex, family history) and those that can (e.g. blood serum cholesterol level, ci, smoking, high blood pressure).

Ed and Rec identified competencies needed by the health educator
1949 First U.S. Office of Ed Conference on Undergrad Professional Prep of Students majoring in health ed directed by HF Kilander

1940's Addition of behavioral science theory and inter-personal process to curriculum Specialities of schools: NC, community org;

Minn. & Mich., school health; UCB, behavioral sci & processes

1950's...

Society of Public Health Educators - Dr. Clair Turner, first president –Fifty charter members

Membership stayed at 500-600 until 1960's

1950 The Nat'l Conference on Graduate Study in Health, PE

and Rec established gui for grad educatio.

Mid-Century –White I Conference on Childr Youth recommended g emphasis of health ed school curriculum t adequately prepared te

1953 Creation of the Department of Hea Education and Welf

PHILOSOPHY OF HEALTH EDUCATION (Adapted from Baelz 1979)

The bedrock of health education is the belief in voluntary participation and empowerment of the learner. It is based on the following philosophy.

Some vision of a healthy society and man's interrelationship, sets health in the context of culture and relates it to human values. The center of our concern thereby moves from the avoidance of pain, distress, dissatisfaction and the elimination of disease to the search for meaning, fulfillment and joy. The Navaho concept of health as symptomatic of a correct relationship between man and his environment represents the 'delicate balance' which a healthy relationship with the total environment requires.

Once we have set health in the context of human values, the nature of health education shifts. Health education must include more than instruction in hygiene and the rules for self-preservation. It must concern itself with values and attitudes, with self-understanding and commitment, with persons in the making.

There are no professionals or experts in the field of human values. Wisdom and authority are widely diffused. In dealing with human values, we are all ordinary men and women, sharing our experiences and insights. The authority of key persons in the community who have wisdom and insight and are influential, cannot be imposed, it has to be acknowledged. It is complementary, not antithetical, to have respect for the individual and his freedom.

Is "changing people's attitudes" incompatible with respecting individual freedom of choice? Yes, if the methods of change are manipulative. Respect for persons rules out manipulation. On the other hand, freedom of choice is not to be equated with choice in a vacuum, which would be an

1954 The School Health Ed Evaluation Study in Los Angeles examines effects of comprehensive school health education	**1958 Inter-Agency Conference on School Health Ed, recommends effective communication among the various elements involved in health ed**	**1960's...** **1961 School Health Ed Study (SHES) surveyed nearly 1 million students nationwide and initiated the writing of a K-12 curriculum directed by E. Sliepcevich**
1956 Two College Health conferences were chaired by Ed. B. Johns; the first analyzed health content and methodology; the second studied professional prep of school health educators	**1959 Highland Park Conf established commissions to study specific issues (philosophy, health instruction, research, intergroup relationships and accreditation)**	**1966 The Committee on Grad Curriculum in Health Ed offered recommendations for a core curriculum that included health science, behavioral science education, and**

arbitrary decision rather than considered choice in accordance with sincerely held values and bel
Freedom of choice should properly be taken to signify self-possession and self-determination.
Freedom of choice is not absolute independence but must be exercised in relationship to others.
cannot help influencing each other's beliefs and attitudes, it is an important part of education. T
difference between education and manipulation lies in the aim of the educator who encourages h
pupil to develop the capacity to think for himself. Eventually the educator will find that he is tal
to an equal, and furthermore, himself often becomes the learner. The process of teaching works
both directions. Thus, in the context of human values health education is never simply imparting
information by the one who knows to the one who does not know. It is a communication of insi
shared exploration of a shared humanity, a venture of "persons in the making."

research

1969 Teach Us What We Want to Know, a needs and interest survey of 5,000 Connecticut students directed by Ruth Byler

1970's...

*Major focus on physician/medical care system - access and cost containment.
Two branches of health education; school health*

education and public health education had grown independently of each other. A dialogue between organizations representing the two branches began to grow

1971 Officially changed title to Society for Public Health Education but retained SOPHE acronym and logo. Stated purpose was: "to promote, encourage and contribute to the health of all

people by encouraging improving practices, elevating standards in th of health education

Strong State Health Edu Programs -CA, PA, NC,

1971 Coalition of Nat Health Education Organizations– Members: AAHE; SSDF ACHA; SOPHE; APHA-PHES; CSTDF

PRINCIPLES OF HEALTH EDUCATION

Participation is a basic principle. People affected by the problem must be involved in defining the problem, planning and implementing steps to resolve the problem and establishing structures to ensure that desired change is maintained. This promotes ownership, meaning that local people must have a sense of responsibility for, and control over, the program, promoting change so they will continue to support the changes. *(Bracht 1990)*

Participation enables the change program to be designed and adapted to the wide range of learning experiences and current circumstances that affect the group. (See also Community Settings section.)

Program design foundations:
The first task in changing behavior is to determine its characteristics by a needs assessment and then systematically develop a variety of interventions as resources allow based on theory, data, and participation. Behavior has multiple bases so we need multiple methods to effect change.

Interventions are educational rather than coercive or manipulative and consist of education, training, resource development, and rewards. First things first. Interventions and their subsumed learning experiences usually have a logical developmental sequence and should build on the experience that the learner already has. As much as possible adapt learning experiences to each individual. When that is not possible in large scale programs, provide self-help and review materials and feedback mechanisms. Immediate feedback helps learners adapt to new ideas.

There is no built in superiority or inferiority in any method of intervention to achieve behavioral change. It depends on the circumstances, the target audience, the timing, the enthusiasm

APHA-SHS; ASHA	Consumer Health Information & Health Promotion Act of 1976	School Health within the Dept of Ed created by PL 95-561
1972 The President's Committee on Health Education under President Nixon. Sub-Committee Patient Education	OHIP Office of the Surgeon General - PHS - HHS	Conference on the Commonalities and Differences in the Preparation and Practice of Health Educators held in Bethesda, MD
	1977 National Center for Health Education	
1974 PL 93-641 National Health Planning & Resources Development Act Federal Focus est. Bureau of Health Education in CDC	1978 National Center for Health Ed facilitated the Role Delineation Project	1979 Healthy People: The Surgeon General's Report on Health Promotion and Disease Prevention
1976 94-317 National	Office of Comprehensive	

and commitment of the change agent. *(Adapted from Green 1991)*

The effectiveness of specific interventions depends on their appropriate selection and application. Predictive of effectiveness are reinforcement, feedback, individualization, facilitatic and relevance. *(Mullen 1990)*

Principles of learning *(Reference unavailable)*
1. Learning is an experience which occurs inside the learner and is activated by the learn
2. Learning is the discovery of the personal meaning and relevance of ideas.
3. Learning (behavioral change) is a consequence of experience.
4. Learning is a cooperative and collaborative process.
5. Learning is an evolutionary process.
6. Learning is sometimes a painful process.
7. The learner himself is one of the richest resources for learning.
8. The process of learning is emotional as well as intellectual.
9. The processes of problem-solving and learning are highly unique and individual.

Conditions which facilitate learning:
A situation that encourages people to be active; promoting individual discovery of the personal meaning of ideas, emphasizes the uniquely personal and subjective nat learning, that difference is good and desirable; that people have a right to make mistakes; display tolerance of ambiguity; a cooperative process with emphasis on self evaluation; encourages open of self; that permits confrontation; that encourage learners to trust themselves as well as external sources; where people feel respected and accepted.

Adult Education Concepts. Andragogy, the art and science of teach adults is based on a set of assumptions about learning that are different from traditional pedagog

---

1980's...
Focus on health promotion/wellness for individuals

1985 The Initial Role Delineation for Health Education, Final Report published

1987 AAHE Directory lists 317 professional preparation programs in school & community health education

1988 Establishment of National Commission for Health Education Credentialing, Inc.

1990's...
Focus on impact of environmental/policy issues on health, and distributive justice

1990 First examination for Certified Health Education

Specialist (CHES)

1990 Healthy People 200 national health promotic prevention priorities. In health education for firs

1991 AAHE Directory lis professional preparat. programs in school communitiy, and public . education

four main assumptions are:

Changes in self-concept- As a person matures his self-concept moves from one of total dependency (as an infant) to increasing self-directedness.

Experience- Increasing use of experiential techniques as the growing reservoir of experience of an adult causes him to be an expanding and richer resource for learning. This conveys a respect for the adult as a unique individual.

Readiness to learn- Assumption that learners are ready to learn those things they " need" because of the development phases that are approaching in their multiple roles. This contrasts with pedagogical approach of providing what "ought" to be learned. The critical implication here is the importance of timing learning experiences to coincide with learners' developmental tasks.

Orientation to learning- The adult's is a problem-centered orientation to learning instead of subject-centered orientation. It differs from a child's learning in that a child's learning is one of postponed application vs. the adult learning emphasis on immediacy of application. *(Knowles 1978)*

NCIPLES

FOR

SSIONAL

ETHICS

GUIDELINES ADOPTED BY THE SOCIETY FOR PUBLIC HEALTH EDUCATION

1. DO NOT DISCRIMINATE AGAINST OTHERS

2. OBSERVE INFORMED CONSENT PRACTICES

3. VALUE PRIVACY, DIGNITY, AND WORTH OF THE INDIVIDUAL

4. MAINTAIN PROFESSIONAL COMPETENCE

5. FOSTER A NURTURING EDUCATIONAL ENVIRONMENT

6. SUPPORT CHANGE BY CHOICE, NOT COERCION

7. HONEST REPORTING OF RESEARCH AND PRACTICE

8. ACT WITHIN BOUNDARIES OF PROFESSIONAL COMPETENCE

9. ACT APPROPRIATELY AT NOTICE OF UNETHICAL PRACTICE

SOME EXAMPLES OF EFFECTIVE
HEALTH EDUCATION

Farquhar, J.W., S.P. Fortmann, J.A. Flora, et al. "Effects of Commu Wide Education on Cardiovascular Disease Risk Factors—The Stanford 5-City Project." JAMA (1990): 359-65.

Puska, P., N. Aulikki, et al. "The Community Based Strategy to Pre Coronary Heart Disease: Conclusions from the Ten Years of the North Karelia Project." An. Re Public Health 6 (1985): 147-93.

Morisky, D.L., D.M. Levine, L.W. Green, et al. "Five-Year Blood Pressure Control and Mortality Following Health Education for Hypertensive Patients." AJPH 7 (1983): 153-62.

Kotchen, J.M., H.E. McKean, S. Jackson-Thayer, et al. "Impact of a High Blood Pressure Control Program on Hypertension Control and Cardiovascular Mortality." JAMA 255 (1986): 2177-82.

Garraway, W.M. and J.P. Whisnant. "The Changing Pattern of Hypertension and the Declining Incidence of Stroke." JAMA 258 (1987): 214-17.

Hersey, J.C., L.S. Klibanoff, D.J. Lam, and R.L. Taylor. "Promoting Support: The Impact of California's 'Friends Can Be Good Medicine' Campaign." Health Educa Quarterly 11 (1984): 293-311.

Bertera, R.L. "Planning and Implementing Health Promotion in the Workplace: A Case Study of the DuPont Company Experience." Health Education Quarterly 17 1990): 307-327.

Grana, J. "Preventive Medicine and Employee Productivity." Harvar Business Review 63 no. 2 (1985): 18-29.

Weinberger, M.J., J.M. Greene and M. Jerin. "Health Beliefs and Sm Behavior." AJPH 71 (1981): 1253-55.

Evans, D., N.M. Clark, C.H. Feldman, et al. "A School Health Educa Program for Children with Asthma Aged 8-11 Years." Health Education Quarterly 14 (Fall 198 267-79.

Simons-Morton, B.G., S. Brink, and D. Bates. "Effectiveness and Co Effectiveness of Persuasive Communications and Incentives in Increasing Safety Belt Use." He Education Quarterly 14, no. 2 (Summer 1987): 167-79.

I NEEDS ASSESSMENT

Key Practice Questions

1. If you were starting an AIDS program and wanted to know which group to target, which statistics would you use a) vital statistics, b) cumulative mortality data, c) age-specific mortality data, d) hospital emergency utilization.

2. A local health department wants you, the health education specialist, to help develop a school based health clinic. The local school board is opposed. Which technique would you use to initiate a productive dialogue? a) focus group, b) Delphi approach, c) nominal group process, d) force field analysis.

3. For an unidentified illness, which records would be most useful? a) school absenteeism, b) health screenings, c) physician's medical records, d) hospital emergency records.

4. The best demographic predictor for success in health education programs is: a) ethnicity, b) age, c) sex, d) educational attainment.

5. The median age of a community is 20.7. Most residents do not complete school past the 7th grade, infant mortality is a big problem. The median age indicates, a) high fertility rate, b) low fertility rate, c) need for community colleges, d) high immigration rate.

. H. E. S.
UIREMENT

1.1, 1.2,   Assess environmental, individual & group characteristics to identify health needs, interests, and concerns
1.3 Assess resources to determine feasibility of health ed program

Needs assessment is a systematic planned collection of information about the reported needs of individuals or groups. It provides the logical starting point for program planning and for action providing the scientific and political base for program planning. It is the basis for sound planning and eliciting participant buy-in. It is basically a data collection endeavor coupled with the process of target group or community participation. It is linked with the process of determining and ranking priorities but is separate and distinct. Needs assessment is an indispensable tool for priority rating, but ultimately, priority determination exercises are colored by political and value judgments.

Needs assessment is an integral part of the program planning process.

One author breaks needs assessment at the community level into analysis and diagnosis: Community analysis is data gathering with the involvement of citizens on the backdrop, health status, health care system and social assistance system. Community diagnosis - synthesis of all information collected to identify gaps or problems between health status and the provision of health services within the area. *(Dignan 1987)*

A. GATHER HEALTH RELATED DATA - Use multiple methods

    1. Sources of Data -
          Community Health Status
              Vital Statistics, Local Records
          Community Health Care System - manpower, service delivery
          Community Social Assistance System
          Geographic and Physical Identifiers
          Business & Commerce
          Demographic Characteristics
          Social, Cultural & Political Structure
          State and Federal
              Records, reportable diseases
              Special Surveys–ex., NHIS, NHHANES,
              Epidemiological Studies
          Literature
    2. Data Collection Tools (See page 26)
          Community
              Resource Inventory
              Social Indicators
              Key Informant Approach
              Community Forum
              Public Hearings
              Structured Groups -focus, nominal, Delphi panel
              Survey - methods and techniques
          School
              Cumulative Record
              Standardized Tests and Psychometric Tests
              Screening
              Interviews (teachers, parents, school nurses)
              Surveys
          Medical Setting
              Hospital Admissions & Discharge Data
              Patient Records
              Community Data (see above)
              Interviews and Surveys
          Worksite
              Health Risk Appraisal/Assessment
              Interviews and Surveys
              Community Data
              Focus Groups

The two types of community analyses are geographical/political and functional.

Geo-political community analysis requires:
1. The map of the service area - political boundaries if applicable
2. Identification and plotting of major health services on the map
3. Total population
4. Age distribution
5. Average household income
6. Main sources of community income
7. Total racial and ethnic distribution in the area
8. Other pertinent information

The functional community analysis requires:
1. Identification of factors that make this a community;
profession ethnicity, work setting or type of condition
2. How can these community members be identified?
3. How can they be accessed in terms of communication?
4. Who are the decision-makers or gatekeepers for this group?

Organizations are important for health educators to analyze and understand and take into account in assessment and planning. First, health services are delivered by them, and health programs are shaped by their requirements and constraints. Second, organizing or providing liaison or building coalitions on an inter-agency basis can be facilitated. Also, health educators with few exceptions are employees whose working environment can promote health and safety or not, and may or may not be amenable to health promotion programs.

Organizational analysis questions:
1. Organization chart (who is in charge? who reports to whom?)
2. Mission of organization and /or statement of philosophy
3. Source of funding
4. Policies of the agency and legal mandates related to your program or project
5. Level of funding for health education
6. Numbers and qualifications of those in charge of health education
7. What are the major health education directions? What health education programs are now in place? Are they competitive/complementary to your plan?
8. At what level will decisions be made about the initiation or continuation of this program?
9. What will be the basis for the decisions about: money? public relations? constituent support? community need?
10. Who are the stakeholders in the status quo? Who would benefit or have a piece of the action if new programs are adopted?
11. Who are (will be) the supporters or the detractors of these ideas?
12. Identify the formal and informal communications channels within the organization

B. ANALYZE INFLUENCES ON HEALTH BEHAVIOR
Knowledge, attitudes, beliefs

Culture, significant others, environmental factors
Power- three kinds: legitimate power, reward power and
coercive power *(French and Raven 1959)*
Skills, access to resources
Economic and environmental impacts
Policies
Theories -See page 101

C. ASSESS RESOURCES INCLUDING BARRIERS AND FACILITATORS
Concerned citizens, stakeholders, competition, collaborators
Community competence, self-help, resource development
Analyze policies, resources, and circumstances in the intra
or interorganizational situation that can hinder or facilitate
Tools -See page26

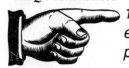

N. C. H. E. S.
REQUIREMENT

1.4 Interpret assessment and summarize assessment by analyzing environmental, individual, and group resource data in order to determine priorities for program development

D. INTERPRET NEEDS FOR HEALTH EDUCATION
Analyze data–epidemiological & statistical concepts
Local estimates based on national/state data
Interpret written, graphic, verbal data - use charts, graphs
Compare to local, state, national data or historical status
Social and attitudinal needs

E. SET PRIORITIES
Criteria: Importance-prevalence, immediacy (urgency),
necessity (must be present for change to occur) changeability

See Hanlon priority list page 25

HANLON PRIORITY METHOD

Components and Criteria to Consider:

A. Size of the Problem

                    Percentage of population directly affected

B. Seriousness of the Problem

                    Urgency - public concern, public health concern

                    Severity - mortality rates; morbidity, degree & duration; disability, degree and duration; accessibility, average distance to care and affordability

                    Medical Costs - individuals directly affected; third party payers

                    Future Needs - potential number who may acquire problem or be affected by problem; relative degree of complication and involvement.

C. Effectiveness of the Solution - How well can the problem be solved?

                    Defined as improvement of the service or programs offered or in relation to current services as a result of the implementation of the suggested solution.

                    CRITERIA CHECKLIST FOR PRIORITIZING HEALTH PROBLEMS *(Hanlon)*

                    A. Percent of Population Affected
                    B. Economical Loss
                    C. Loss of Manpower (productivity)
                    D. Severity
                    E. Urgency
                    F. Medical Costs
                    G. Future Need
                    H. Economic Feasibility
                    I. How Easily Can We Solve This Problem
                    J. How Quickly Can We Solve This Problem
                    K. Are There Enough Resources
                    L. Legality
                    M. Acceptability
                    N. Priority

PEARL is an acronym used to remember the Hanlon priorities. It stands for **P**riority, **E**conomic Feasibility, **A**cceptability, **R**esources, **L**egality.

NEEDS ASSESSMENT TOOLS

Surveys Complex and expensive. Use to get knowledge, attitudes, beliefs, behavior. G
survey is well constructed, tested for validity, has high response rate and valid sample. Surveys
reactive and may arouse expectations. Survey formats are mail (cheapest, may have low respons
rate, only for literate, info is structured & limited), telephone (faster, selective to those with pho
more depth possible), face-to-face (expensive, can get in-depth responses). Data analysis and rep
dissemination should be planned at outset.

Unstructured or moderately structured interviews Pros: More opportunity than sur
to discover information, obtain more complete info, especially suited for obtaining valuable info
busy people. Cons: Interviewers need knowledge of the subject of interview (the less interviewe
background, the more structured the interview and more training is needed), data analysis is mor
difficult; they are more costly.

Key informant interviews Key informants are strategically placed individuals who ha
knowledge and ability to report on the needs of an institution, if you are working in a corporatio
hospital, or in the community. They are aware of the needs and services perceived by the target
important. Because they are important members, they can affect the support and buy-in for prog
changes. They may be biased. The full range of community perspective should be reflected in
selection. The "snowball" technique where they are asked to recommend others for interviews ca
provide insights into networks and communicators. Key informant surveys are quick and relative
inexpensive to conduct. Ten to 15 questions maximum should cover both general and specific ne
target population, issues of accessibility and acceptability of solutions. Recommend mail or phor
notice which includes outline of questions and a face-to-face interview.

Resource inventories Use of records and agency interviews can establish who is provi
services, what services are provided, comprehensiveness and continuity of service, and where
problems and gaps exist.

Observational methods for large scale studies Outcomes of the target population are
measured directly rather than indirectly through self-reports or reports of others. Most of the
techniques listed assume that direct observational information is not available or relevant. Like
epidemiological surveys, most observational techniques are complicated and require expert
consultation.

Community forums A public meeting seeking broad scale participation in order to rev
various perspectives on a particular subject. Pros: Relatively straightforward to conduct, relativ
inexpensive, opportunity for all views since it is publicly advertised; people can participate on th
own terms; can identify people who are most interested and may later be prepared to participate.
hard to generate attendance, draws respondents with special interests; can degenerate into gripe
session, data analysis may be time consuming.

Electronic conferencing Alternative to face-to-face meetings, video, audio, computer teleconferencing slow to develop because of cost and discomfort of participants. Audio less expensive than video but requires more discipline on part of paricipant to listening and how to contribute. Pros: Way to bring widely scattered people together are relatively low cost; way to bring busy people together; can be conducted relatively quickly; individuals not influenced by status differences. Cons: Interaction limited, for participants who are highly verbal, requires access to technology, costly.

Force field analysis Diagramming of a problem based on the assumption that any situation is a temporary balance between opposing forces. The driving forces facilitating change and those restraining change are identified and rated according to their importance forces by drawing arrows on diagram below to weight the strength of the force according to analyzer perception. Strategies for changing the most important resisting forces or strengthening facilitators are developed according to these goal setting criteria: **S** -Specificity. Exactly what are you trying to accomplish? **P** - Performance. What behavior is implied? **I** -Involvement. Who is going to do it? **R** -Realism. Can it be done? **O** -Observability. Can others see the behavior? The acronym **SPIRO** can aid your thought process

Figure 6
ORCE FIELD
ANALYSIS
_ist the forces
that tend to
support the
status quo
and then list
the forces
that push
>ward change

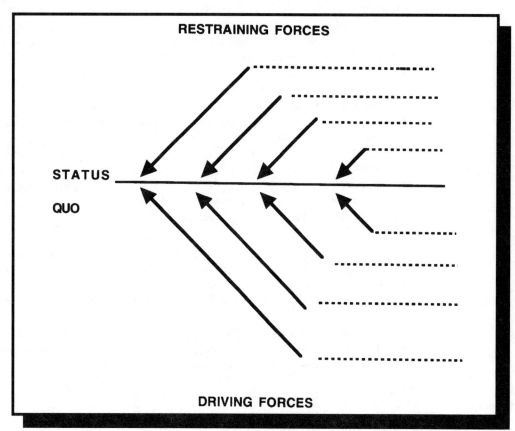

RESTRAINING FORCES

STATUS

QUO

DRIVING FORCES

STRUCTURED GROUPS

Nominal Group Process Allows for idea generation and evaluation while avoiding the problems of group dynamics. Overcomes problem of a few individuals dominating the discussion. Requires room large enough for all participants, tables for 6-9, flip chart, and index cards. Takes hours.

Steps: 1) Develop questions for participants requiring differentiated solutions; 2) Break groups should represent all perspectives in large group; 3) Participants answer question by writing cards, no discussion allowed; 4) Ideas are recorded on flip chart in round robin; 5)Explanation and clarification then encouraged but no criticism or collapsing; 6) Each group member privately rank ideas (e.g. top five). Cards handed in and recorded on flip chart; 7) Brief clarifying discussion; 8) Private ranking again by each member and rankings from all subgroups combined for overall tally. Cycle repeated for each question or issue.

Focus Group Process Small group discussion with structured and open-ended questions. Sampling purposive, not random, to represent target population perspective. Similar to open-ended interviews but responses are not independent. However, allows for quicker data collection. If results are at variance with expectations based on other need identification techniques, additional data collection may be required. Useful for formative evaluation and program/materials development.

Delphi Panels A form of group process that generates a consensus through a series of questionnaires. Usually the respondents are unable to meet in one place due to geographical or limitations. It is used as a forecasting technique and also to clarify, prioritize, or identify problems and solutions. Process involves three groups: decision-makers, staff, and respondent group. Sometimes the decision-makers and the staff are the same group. A questionnaire consisting of two broad questions is sent to the respondents. Their responses are analyzed and from these, a second questionnaire is developed. More specific questions for further clarification are included, their responses are again analyzed and another questionnaire is sent out asking for additional information. The usual number of rounds is three to five.

Pros: appropriate when accurate info not available; people separated by geography can be involved (often the experts); conformity, domination, or conflict is reduced since no face-to-face; written responses encourage quality and quantity; ideas given equal representation; usually highly committed individuals; feedback enables participants to respond throughout process and have a sense of closure at end.

Cons: large amount of administrative time and cost; less opportunity to clarify meaning specifics; no opportunity for dialogue and interaction; considerable time commitment for participants; less reward for respondents who must be highly committed.

INDIVIDUAL ASSESSMENT

      Health Risk Appraisal/Assessment (HRA)– describes an individual's chance of becoming ill or dying from a particular cause over a period of time. Not a traditional medical appraisal for detection and identification of disease but a statement of probability. It is based on a comparison with mortality statistics and epidemiological data and is focused on behavior and personal characteristics. Demonstrates relationship between certain risk factors and specific causes of death or disability. It is intended to raise individual level of awareness/knowledge of personal risk factors and potential health outcomes; serve as a vehicle for health education counseling in order to promote voluntary health-related behavior change; serve as group needs assessment instrument for planning health education/health promotion programs. Often computerized. Privacy and confidentiality is a critical issue in worksite settings where this tool is usually used. It is useful also for adult health promotion programs in other settings.

      Checklist Needs Assessment– a list of topics that potential participants check to indicate interest. Easy to administer and tally and clients seldom object. Problem is that checklists usually reflect what professionals are ready to teach, not necessarily the interests of patients. Useful if carefully constructed. Leave space for "other," include topics from both patients and professionals, use focus group for construction.

STEPS IN DESIGNING AND COMPLETING A SURVEY *(Dever 1991)*

1. Determine the objectives. Be sure to consult with those who have interests o outcomes at stake (the stakeholders).

2. Define the population groups to be studied.

3. Determine the specific data to be collected and the methods of measuremen

4. Choose the sampling unit and the sample size.

5. Determine the method of contacting individuals–interview, mailed question telephone? Plan methods to reduce non-response rates.

6. Construct the questionnaire to obtain the desired information. Use existing validated items when possible. Field test.

7. Organize and carry out the interviews. Hire, train and manage interviewers Determine how refusals and non responses will be handled.

8. Process and analyze the data. This includes coding, keypunching, tabulating selecting appropriate statistical methods to specify relationships and significance.

9. Report the results. These should include implications and recommendation: actions.

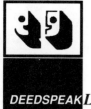

DEEDSPEAK
Author
Comment *Lack of an adequate survey design guarantees failure!*

II PLAN EFFECTIVE HEALTH EDUCATION PROGRAMS

1. What is the most important component of a health promotion program aimed at lowering cholesterol? a) blood cholesterol measurements on all participants, before, during & after program; b) lowering fat intake; c) proper food selection & preparation; d) having an RD on staff.

2. If you were just starting a new health promotion program, which group would you work with? a) journalists; b) local health officials; c) a community based organization (CBO); d) doctors & nurses.

3. What's the first step in a behavioral diagnosis? a) identifying predisposing factors; b) listing enabling factors; c) identifying the barriers to change; d) selecting the health problem to be analyzed.

4. Two major factors of the Health Belief Model are: a) beliefs about perceived seriousness and causal attribution; b) belief in susceptibility and belief in benefits of treatment; c) cues to action and dissonance reduction; d) unfreezing and refreezing.

5. Reciprocal determinism in Social Learning Theory posits: a) continuing adaptation and change between a person, his behavior, and the environment; b) a stage of precontemplation before change; c) the perception or belief in a person's ability to perform; d) occurrences independent of your action that make you feel helpless.

6. In the PRECEDE model, which of the factors in the educational diagnosis deals with the support functions of parents, and/or health providers? a) enabling, b) predisposing, c) reinforcing, d) communicating.

7. Operant conditioning is a useful technique for: a) reducing cognitive dissonance; b) planning a clinic screening; c) helping select individuals maintain weight-loss diets; d) improving physical fitness.

8. At the completion of the program, 70% of the students in ABC School District will improve their physical fitness by 25%. Select the correct response: a) this is formative evaluation; b) this is an impact objective; c) this is a goal statement, d) this is a process objective.

9. At the completion of the instruction, 85% of the participants will select at least ten correct answers to 12 questions on hypertension. In community health planning this is: a) a process objective; b) a behavioral objective; c) an impact objective; d) an outcome objective.

10. Within five years of the initiation of the program, the adults in Mohawk County will attain

the national average of 1.8 dental visits per year. This is: a) a complete behavioral obj~
b) an incomplete behavioral objective; c) a complete program objective; d) an incomple~
program objective.

11. Following are four levels of objectives to be accomplished in an unwanted pregnan~
reduction program: A. self esteem and assertiveness will be increased by 20% in 400 ~
and 8th grade females within 8 months; B. the infant mortality rate among women und~
residing in Census tracts X will be reduced by 15% by 1995; C use of contraception by
sexually active males and females in Louville, U.S.A. will increase by 60% as measure~
self-reports; D rates of pregnancy among females in 9th and 10th grade in View Schoo~
District will be reduced by 56% in two years. Select the developmental sequence that
indicates which objectives must be accomplished first, second, third, fourth in order to ~
the program objective a) ACDB, b) BDCA, c) DCAB, d) ABCD.

DEFINITION - Planning is the process of establishing priorities, diagnosing c~
of problems, and allocating resources to achieve objectives.

The implication of planning is that social problems are remedial in ways
are generally acceptable to those affected by them.

Planning and evaluation for health must take into account the entire fabr~
society and its institutions—in essence, the community. *(Dever 1991)*

Planned change is an intended, designed, or purposive attempt by an
individual, group, organization or larger social system to influence directly the ~
quo of itself, another organism or situation. *(Lippett 1978)*

The definitions, methods, and concepts of community organization can ~
applicable to a school, corporation, or medical care settings as well as communi~
Additional definitions and concepts can be found in the community settings sec~
"A community is a group of people with some things in common who a~

N. C. H. E. S. aware of those commonalities." *(Breckon 1989)*

REQUIREMENT

*2.1 Collaborate with community agencies and individuals by coordinati~
resources and services*
*2.2 Collaborate with potential participants by involving them in plan
development*

2.1-2 COLLABORATE- Communicate a shared vision. Involve and mobilize target groups, significant others, resources. In school health programs, the collaboration is usually with parents. Analyze who has positive and negative stake in change (stakeholders). Analyze power in organization or community—location and degree.

Strategies for acceptance *(Craig 1978)*

1. Explain why the reason for changing. 2. Name the benefits that could result from the change. 3. Seek questions and answer them. 4. Invite participation. 5. Avoid surprise.
6. Acknowledge the rough spots. 7. Set standards (date for completion, what you want change to accomplish, identify penalties for failure, rewards for success). 8 Contact leaders. 9. Praise - give positive reinforcements. 10. Repeat - tell story over and over with fresh examples.

. H . E . S .
UIREMENT

2.3 Develop the health education plan to meet health needs by applying theory and integrating assessment data, community resources and services and input from potential participants.

2.3 THEORY

The PRECEDE model is a useful framework for planning. *(Green, et al 1980)* It focuses on outcomes rather than starting with inputs, identifying specific educational steps to be completed in more detail than the Sullivan model. The steps are epidemiological and social diagnoses, behavioral diagnosis, educational and environmental diagnosis, and administrative diagnosis.

An additional step called PROCEED has been added to the administrative diagnosis in the newest edition of this model. *(Green & Kreuter 1991)* This extends the consideration of **P**olicy, **R**egulatory and **O**rganizational barriers that could facilitate or hinder the development of the educational or environmental program during the implementation phase. Applying PROceed at the behavioral and environmental diagnostic phase (Phase 3) or the MATCH model *(Simons-Morton)* while planning is also important to determine whether your target for the educational diagnosis should be, (for example,) policy makers, resource allocators, or parents rather than those who manifest the problem.

The PRECEDE model is also used to plan educational programs in organizational settings such as worksite, medical care, and schools. The organization's mission may impinge on the goals and objectives of your plan. (See the Needs Assessment section page 21 for additional comments about organizational analysis.)

Organization development (OD) is the application of a long-range planned-change technology to improve problem-solving and renewal processes by means of which an organization changes its culture. Two of the OD methods particularly useful for health educators are team building and conflict management. *(Ross 1984)*

2.3 DEVELOP A PLAN

Plan for the plan. Analysis of your own agency. (See page 21 Needs Assessment) Logical scope and sequence.

Program planning is based on written plans which include the following elements: pro goals, measurable objectives, appropriate activities, description of resources necessary evaluation procedures. <u>Evaluation procedures are developed prior to program implementation</u> <u>and included in the written program plan.</u> *(Standards of Practice 1991)*

Sullivan's steps in planning are process and stress the importance of participation begi with 1) involve people, 2) set goals, 3) define problems and issues, 4) design the program, 5) implement plans, 6) evaluate.

Use the PRECEDE MODEL to formulate a more specific educational plan by carryin social, epidemiological, and behavioral diagnoses. Select a minimum of three strategies based predisposing, reinforcing, and enabling factors. *(Green, et al)*

2.3 FORMULATE APPROPRIATE AND MEASURABLE PROGRAM OBJECTIVES

Written objectives communicate to all other persons the direction and intent of the pla

Check list for objectives
• Objectives should be clear statements.
• Objectives should include just one indicator.
• Objectives should state reasonable time frames.
• Outcome objectives should be stated as performance, not effort.
• Objectives should be realistic and within the control of those responsible.
• Qualities of an objective: relevant, logical, unequivocal, feasible, observable, measu

Use the PRECEDE MODEL to carry out social diagnosis, epidemiological diagnosis, behavioral diagnosis. Select a minimum of three strategies based on predisposing, reinforcing, enabling factors, and use them to write your learning objectives. *(Green, et al 1980)*

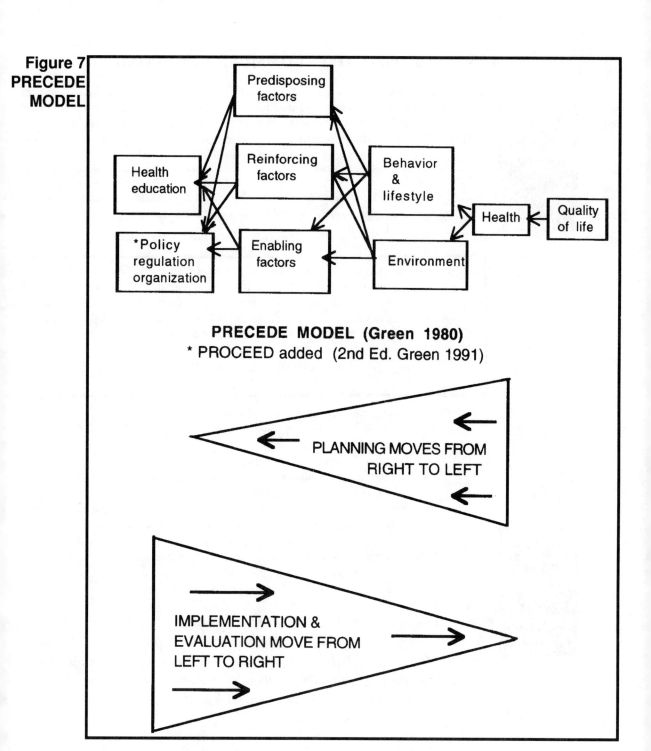

Figure 7
PRECEDE
MODEL

PRECEDE MODEL (Green 1980)
* PROCEED added (2nd Ed. Green 1991)

PLANNING MOVES FROM RIGHT TO LEFT

IMPLEMENTATION & EVALUATION MOVE FROM LEFT TO RIGHT

LEVELS OF OBJECTIVES COMMUNITY PLANNING

Goal or mission statement. A broad timeless statement of long-range program purpose . should summarize the elements of the problem statement in positive outcomes and shoul include the health problem or issue to be changed and the target population. It is related to epidemiological and social diagnosis in PRECEDE.

DEEDSPEAK
Author
Comment
Warning! There is a lot of semantic confusion in this area. A number of people interchange the words "goals" and "objectives". These definitions are based on agreement of the authors who are referenced under this section.

Program objectives. Objectives are related to the goal but are specific, measurable stateme of what we want to accomplish at a given point in time (Usually 3-5 years). One or two usu cover your goals. They are **outcome** or future oriented, and related to health status. It is specific statement of the health problem reflected in the social and epidemiological phases PRECEDE and include the following elements:
WHO will do
HOW MUCH of **WHAT** by
WHEN?

• Specify your target population in more detail

• Select target of intervention
   Influence governments for resources & policy changes
   Influence community or organizations for resources, policy and social norms
      changes; to reach influentials
   Influence gatekeepers/influentials to reach/train etc. groups, provide reinforc
   Influence individuals for behavior change or social support

• Identify several strategies to accomplish each objective: e.g.
   media, community organization, formal instruction, social
   support, training for providers, reinforcements, rewards

DEEDSPEAK
Author
Comment
Note: formal instruction is only one strategy and <u>alone</u> is not considered suffic community education strategy It may be viable for school classrooms, some workplace programs, for some patient education classes, for training providers difficult to get people to sit still. Think of all the other ways that people get information and discuss and experiment with health issues in their daily lives selecting several other interventions.

The use of focus groups as a formative evaluation measure is very useful at this juncture. The key to their value is the selection of participants and the types of questions that are posed. The technique provides target group perceptions and emotions in informal group discussions related to the issue. It provides you with useful clues about messages, types of interventions, new viewpoints.

> **Impact objectives** describe the behaviors or actions that will resolve the problem and get you to your program goal. (Usually 1-3 years). They are also written as Who will do How Much of What by When. In the PRECEDE model this phase is called the Behavioral Diagnosis.

Evaluation planning starts here while you are drafting program and impact objectives. Think about how you will tell when the change has taken place? What will people be doing that they aren't doing now?

What is the indicator or measure that you will use to measure your success? By adding this now, your evaluation steps are already evolving.

> **Add measurement criteria to your objectives** with a sentence specifying indicators. (How can we tell that there has been a change—how much change is needed to be acceptable?)

Identify the percentage of change (the number of participants or the amount of an observed action). Objectives should articulate those outcomes which must be accomplished to make the program worth the effort and expense. Think about:

How much change will make any noticeable difference?
How difficult will it be to affect change?
How much change has been reported in studies of similar programs?
How expensive or elaborate is the program?
What is the current level of the indicator to be changed?

Process or learning objectives are the educational or learning tasks that must be accompli[...]
to achieve the impact objectives of the intervention. They are based on the analysis o[...]
predisposing, reinforcing, and enabling factors in the PRECEDE model and are specified[...]
knowledge changes, attitude and belief changes, behaviors and skills that are required of[...]
target group or surrounding persons—parents, teachers, peers, providers, reporters, voters,[...]
These make up the daily delivery of the educational activities and are subject to adjustme[...]
they are tested. They are usually short term but can have longer time spans depending upo[...]
design of the program.

Process or administrative objectives are the daily tasks and workplans that lead to[...]
accomplishment of all of your planned objectives.

Table 2
EVELS OF
JECTIVES
OUTPUTS

Objective	Outcome	Evaluation
A. GOAL	Ameliorate Health Problem	Changeability Feasibility
B. PROGRAM OBJECTIVE	Outcome-change in morbidity, mortality, quality of life	Health Change Attributable to Program?
C. ACTION/BEHAVIORAL OBJECTIVE	Impact -Behavioral Adaptation	Action or Desired Behavior? Attributable to Health Education Program?
D. PROCESS/LEARNING OBJECTIVES	Process - Change in Knowledge Attitude Practices	Measures of change Knowledge, Habit, Attitude, Skill, etc.
E. PROCESS/ADMINIS-TRATIVE OBJECTIVES	Activities/Tasks on Schedule, Efficiently	Exposure, Attendance Materials, Schedules, Participation, etc.

When you plan, move from the big idea down to the daily tasks–from the abstract to the concrete. When you implement you start at the opposite end with the daily concrete activities and move up to the more abstract generalized objectives. Moving from the concrete to the bigger, more abstract concepts is also true of evaluation.

The questions that you ask at the process level after your start up are: is the program working? are people coming to the event? listening to the radio?, etc. If they are exposed, are they learning? Or if you are training, are the trainees displaying new skills? Do your clients understand the material? At the learning process level the question is are the methods we chose working? Can we detect changes in attitudes, skills, knowledge? Are we doing the best we can with our resources? Or should we change our methods and try to improve?

At the behavioral or impact level the evaluation question is one of efficacy. Can the action or behavior that will affect the health problem be detected? Can it be attributed to our program?

Curriculum objectives and goals in School Health

Goals are statements of broad intent that provide direction in making instructional decisions—long-range targets toward which instruction is directed. They are more general than objectives and are timeless. Objectives are short-term precise statements of end results that build cumulatively toward a goal and in turn a topic or generalization. Effective complete objectives have a content dimension and a behavioral dimension. Precision in formulating and stating objectives can contribute to more effective teaching. The range of behaviors for learners in school health educa[tion] curriculum should center around the general areas of information acquisition, skill development, concept development, opinion expression and development, and values awareness. *(Fodor 1989)*

**Figure 8
RELATIONSHIP
OF
INSTRUCTIONAL
BEHAVIORAL
OBJECTIVES TO
COMMUNITY
HEALTH
PROGRAM
OBJECTIVES**

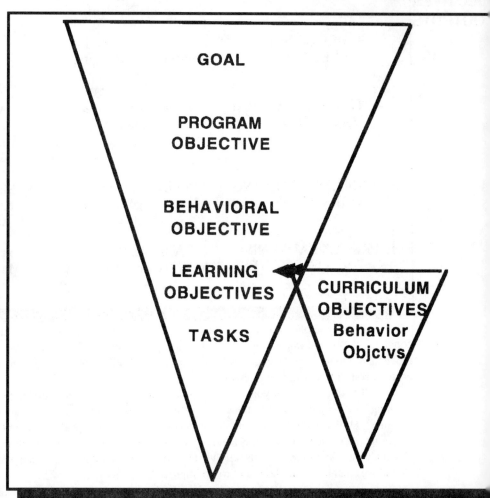

Note: Behavioral objectives in writing curriculum are considered an activity or process objective in community health education planning. Successful learning result in observable behaviors but at this level seldom resolve health problems. Mager's historical book which defined behavioral or measurable objectives was describing curriculum objectives in programmed instruction. Don't confuse them with the behaviors sought at the impact level which aim to reduce health problem[s]

2.3 DESIGN EDUCATIONAL PROGRAMS CONSISTENT WITH OBJECTIVES

The first questions to be asked in selecting strategies and designing an educational program for community health are: what specific behaviors must the learners acquire or enhance to reduce the effect of the problem; what information and skills must be gained in order for them to act in a new way or maintain an existing way; what resources are needed; what related services or other kinds of conditions are required; and, of all the desired changes, which actual actions can be addressed in the educational program.

Methods must be applied, or activities must be performed in order to accomplish the short-term objectives. This program planning defines content, methods, time allotments, materials, facilitators or instructors, etc. A complete set of methods or process objectives constitute a workplan for the program. These activities are inputs that specify a time frame and a target group and they then refer to something the target group will receive or do.

These processes make up the objectives that are monitored, adjusted, or redesigned during the process evaluation stage. (See Section III – Implementation page 45 for detail.) Tasks are related to activities and refer to management or administrative tasks that the agency or personnel must do.

From the activities or tasks, personnel assignments, budgets, and timeplans, personnel responsibilities evolve that must be recorded and monitored to manage the project.

"In school education the behaviors are cognitive and affective performance. Behaviors are focused on 'didn't know how to do, and now can do.' This is the acceptable level of behavior in curriculum objectives." *(M. Pollock)*

Sullivan's Steps in Community Planning *(Sullivan 1973)*

These reflect community health plannning.

1. Involve People *
> Identify persons affected & those who have needed skills
> Determine roles and relationships
> Establish links with persons in related programs

> * Initiation of project is critical to success

2. Set Goals
> Set ultimate goals related to health status, lifestyle, health practices. This is a
> general statement based on vision, quality of life, model standards, etc. Also
> to health educator's agency/sponsor mission statement.

3. Define Problems or Issues
> Determine health status gaps & trends caused by health-related behavior
> Describe characteristics of affected persons–trends in these characteristics
> Analyze positive/negative forces affecting health actions
> Determine gaps, trends, forces regarding health ed resources
> Formulate program focus–aspects of the problems that can and should be tack
> regarding health, action, education resources and forces. Write goal statemen
> outcome

4. Design Program
> List alternative approaches to problem & moving toward goals
> Analyze pros and cons of alternatives in relation to specific criteria
> Select tentative approach (strategy)
> Set specific operational objectives
> Define specific sub-objectives for program & for administration, activities, ti
> and resources
> Pretest and revise plans
> Develop internal and external marketing strategy
> Develop specific evaluation procedures, monitoring, and tracking
> Obtain approvals of plans and commitments of resources

5. Implement Plans
> Obtain needed funds
> Expand involvement to more levels of community activity
> Obtain needed staff, volunteers, committees, and consultants
> Define specific duties and relationships
> Obtain needed facilities, equipment, supplies, and services
> Develop management policies and procedures

Implement plans

Monitor, track for impact, revise, recycle to objectives if necessary

6. Evaluate (see Section IV – Evaluation page 49)

PRELIMINARY NOTES FOR THE PLANNER

Plan with people

Plan with data

Plan for permanence—staff time most expensive ingredient

Plan for priorities

Plan for outcomes and impact

Plan for evaluation

Plan for the plan

Who should be involved

Data needed

Best time to plan

Where it should occur

Anticipate resistances

What will enhance success of project

Timetable (*Gantt or Pert Chart, see page 48*)

EVALUATION PLANNING IS PART OF PROGRAM DESIGN

After answering the questions that are noted at the beginning of Section 2.3 Designing Educational Programs, continue the raising of questions to articulate the evaluation issues: what actions or behaviors can and should you try to measure; what specific measures will be used and when; what educational techniques or methods are best and how can you monitor them; do you to plan training for agency staff or for program personnel; what organizational resources or arrangements are needed; what budget is required; is your organization able and willing to provi required resources?

Pre-implementation Checklist: *(Forouzesh 1991)*

1. Clearly determine who does what, for whom, in what order, by when, and with what resources.

2. Develop and translate existing policies and procedures.

3. Assess required resources and their sources.

4. Determine and delegate administration and management responsibilities.

5. Develop an efficient communication network.

6. List all steps required and the order in which they must occur.

7. Determine when (date) each step should begin and end.

8. Identify internal and external constraints and factors that facilitate and support the implementation process such as policy-makers, parents, etc.

9. Make sure to monitor and reconfirm the commitment of all those involved in the pro

10. Design monitoring and tracking process to evaluate success of activities and need adjustment or re-design if it isn't working. (see Section IV – Evaluation page 49)

11. Develop a contingency "what if" plan based on what can go wrong, will!

12. Identify implications and the impact of your program on other programs.

13. Identify the most crucial and important steps and activities to complete your progr

III IMPLEMENT THE HEALTH EDUCATION PROGRAM

Key Practice Questions

1. Your program for Vietnamese health promotion is not working. You need additional data. The least expensive and most effective method is: a) random household survey; b) mailed, self-administered questionnaire; c) telephone survey; d) focus group interviews.

2. At the AIDS Taskforce meeting, a professional member of the group asks you a specific question about how the virus works in the body. You have recently read this information, but don't remember the details. Your most professional response is: a) tell the person what you remember; b) give the person the national clearinghouse number; c) say "That's a medical question. Ask Dr. Lego who is sitting over there."; d) say "I have some material on that question which I can mail to you."

3. You have invited representatives of organizations to a meeting to talk about health needs in a neighborhood that has a series of divisive issues. You would like to avoid a conclusion that represents the narrow point of view of a few who speak loudly and may not reflect the whole community. As the responsible staff member, what is the best way to insure community-wide views are represented? a) Add additional representatives and increase participation; b) supplement the proceedings with a community survey; c) label the committee as an ad hoc task group so that its existence can be limited; d) try to keep the group as small as possible.

4. You anticipate divisive advocacy at the above meeting. In order to meet your problem solving and priority setting objectives, the best meeting procedure is: a) close the meeting to media representatives; b) use parliamentary rules with a formal agenda; c) use nominal group process; d) divide into focus groups.

. H. E. S.

UIREMENT

3.1 Implement the health education plan by employing health education methods and techniques in order to achieve program objectives

DEFINITION: Implementation is a systematic approach to putting decisions into the action phase or simply to put a designed plan into action.

Criteria for implementation: *(Standards of Practice 1991)*
Implementation is based on activities and timeliness developed in written plan; it is monitored for necessary adjustments; it includes close collaboration with community groups and leaders.

Before implementing, address the following issues: 1. Is this program acceptable to the target population? 2. Are there adequate resources available to assure the continuation of the program? 3. Is this program legal and do you have the authority to deliver this program?

A SELF STUDY GUIDE FOR PROFESSIONAL COMPETENCE

Processes

1. Planning, conducting, attending meetings
   Purpose of meeting–representation of attendees
   Objectives–selection of format
   Roles = presider, discussion leader, participant
   Skills–summarize, keep discussion on track, encourage participation
   parliamentary procedure for formal discussion
2. Group dynamics
   Facilitate group cohesiveness, decision making, problem solving, sha
   leadership
   Facilitate cooperation and feedback
   Liaison between individuals or group and outside
   Assist in problem analysis and alternative solutions
   Assist in understanding of issues
3. Monitoring program activities
   Develop record system for feedback
   Revise activities based on process evaluation
4. Manage project or program
   Job descriptions, hire, supervise, evaluate personnel
   Monitor budget expenditures
   Develop time plans and task objectives
   Regular reporting to executive board, funder, etc.
   Public relations & marketing strategies (See Section VII – Communi
   page 65)
5. Build participation and trust with target groups & agencies

Table 3

EXAMPLE OF IMPLEMENTATION WORKSHEET FOR ACTIVITIES

Once you have identified the processes to be accomplished, use a worksheet to identify all of the daily tasks and timetables required to reach those objectives. *This sheet can be translated into a Gantt or Pert chart. See Figures 9 & 10. on page 48.*

Resources:

Schedules, deadlines, etc.

Activities	Who does what?	When?
1.		
2.		
3.		
4.		
5.		
6.		
etc.		

Figure 9
TIME AND TASK PLAN OR GANTT CHART

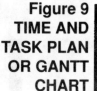

TASK	JAN 6-12	FEB 18-24	MAR 30-36	APR 42-48	MAY 54-60	JUNE 66 72	JULY 78	AUG 84	SE 90.96.102
Contact 8 Sr. Citizen Centers	_ _ _ _								
Plan community meeting for organizations		_ _ _ _							
Plan media campaign		_ _ _ _ _ _							
Develop materials		_ _ _ _ _ _ _ _ _							
Plan and pre-test training for vols.		_ _ _ _ _ _ _ _ _							
Recruit volunteers				_ _ _ _ _ _ _				
Train volunteers					_ _ _ _ _ _ _ _				
Implement campaign							_ _ _ _ _ _ _ _ _		
Report							X		X

Figure 10
PROGRAM EVALUATION & REVIEW TECHNIQUE (PERT)

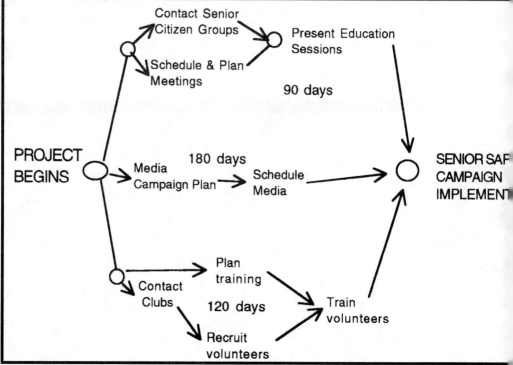

IV EVALUATE EFFECTIVENESS OF HEALTH ED PROGRAMS

Key Practice Questions

1. Performance evaluation and review technique is: a) an evaluation model by Rossi; b) a planning technique suited to groups to set deadlines and schedules; c) an indispensable management tool for small projects; d) a list of all the tasks and personnel assignments.

2. The best time to plan an evaluation is: a) when writing objectives for the overall program; b) when beginning the implementation phase; c) just as soon as the implementation phase is underway; d) 6 months before the program is completed.

3. Cost effectiveness is: a) the cheapest way to achieve the objective;`b) a measure of cost of intervention vs. relative to its benefit; c) cost of intervention relative to its impact; d) the intervention having the most change.

4. Following are four analyses of the perceived benefit of a health education program vs. the effort invested:

		Benefit	
		High	Low
Effort	High	A	C
	Low	B	D

Select the sequence which indicates the most efficient to the least efficient:
a) BADC; b) ABCD; c) CDBA; d) BDAC

5. Focus group input to develop messages for a blood pressure control program is an example of: a) formative evaluation; b) summative evaluation; c) criterion referenced testing; d) monitoring process.

6. Comparison of baseline blood pressure control levels to follow-up survey measures after a two-year intervention is completed is: a) a process evaluation; b) an impact evaluation; c) a formative evaluation; d) an outcome evaluation.

7. A determination that all members of an HMO should maintain blood pressure control measures of 140/90 or below is an example of: a) a criterion-referenced measure; b) a norm-referenced measure; c) a theoretical standard; d) a summative evaluation.

8. If you were analyzing data on numbers of welfare families in cities in the state of New York, including New York City, which descriptive statistic would be more valid: a) mean; b) median; c) mode; d) standard deviation.

10. Pick the one incorrect phrase. Random sampling means that: a) experimental and control groups differ from one another only by self-selection; b) minimizes systematic bı assigned groups; c) every person in the universe has an equal chance to be selected; c makes generalization from your sample to other groups possible.

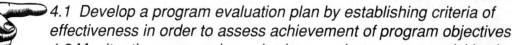

N. C. H. E. S.
REQUIREMENT

4.1 Develop a program evaluation plan by establishing criteria of effectiveness in order to assess achievement of program objectives
4.2 Monitor the program by reviewing ongoing program activities in order determine if the program is being implemented as planned
4.3 Monitor by comparing results with outcome criteria in order to determ program effectiveness
4.4 Modify program as indicated by comparison of results with criteria in order to enhance the likelihood of program success

I EVALUATION PLANNING

See comments under planning which refer to the relationship of program objectives to evaluat See attached table of relationships between PRECEDE, planning objectives, evaluation leve measurements. (Page 51)

• Evaluation is making a judgment based on comparison for the purposes of feedback t improve the quality of human services. Usual standards of comparison are historical (before & a comparison with a group that has not had the intervention; or comparison with standards or norn from national data or theoretical outcomes from the literature.

• Difference between research and evaluation - research addresses issues of theoretical interest without regard for immediate concerns of organizations or people; evaluation generates information related to decision-making, and is done under time constraints. Research tools of va degrees of rigor are used in evaluation

•The purpose of evaluation is to answer one of two questions:

a. "Are we doing the best we can with the resources that we have?"
That is, are we using our resources efficiently—can we change our methods, materials, program to be more effective? EFFICIENCY. This is process evaluation.

b. "Is the program/intervention having any effect?" That is, are any changes that are observed the result of our program? This is called EFFICACY. This is impact evaluat

c. There actually is a third question, "So what?" This question asks if the successful ch made any difference in health status identified as the program goal. Changes in health are outcome evaluation. This is a longer range question, requiring more resources and time and is usually not dealt with by entry-level health educators. However, it is important to keep the question in front of you as a compass.

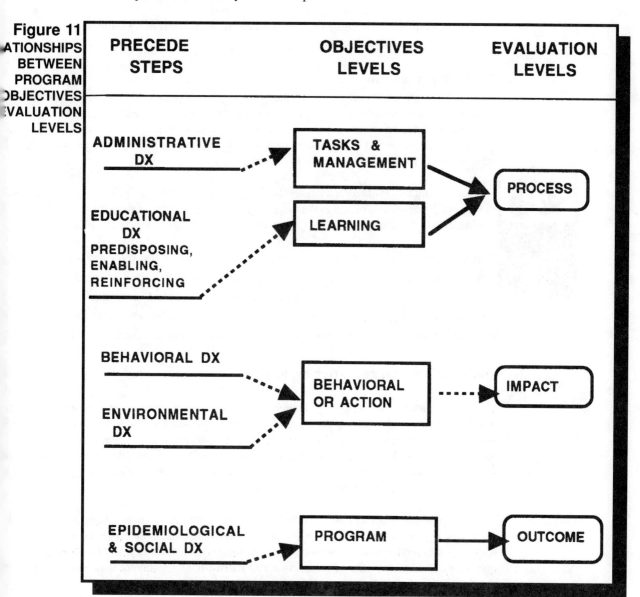

Figure 11
RELATIONSHIPS BETWEEN PROGRAM OBJECTIVES EVALUATION LEVELS

The three levels of evaluation objectives: link back to program objectives
   a. Process - something changes as a result of planned learning and
       management activities
   b. Impact - the intervention leads to an observable action/behavior that
       will have an impact on the health status
   c. Outcomes - action/behavioral adaptation (b) leads to an improvement
       in health status

Types of Evaluation

Formative and **summative** evaluation. These descriptors identify the **purpose or rol** the evaluation and do not refer to methods. Formative evaluation is ongoing improvement in a intervention, program or curriculum. It is done with the explicit purpose of making midstream alterations in the program in order to increase the likelihood of achieving the overall objective. other words, to maximize the success of the intervention.

Summative evaluation assesses the extent to which a finished product or program caus changes in the desired direction in the target population and is justification for the expense of continuation in the present site and/or adoption in other settings. *(DeFriese 1983)*

DEEDSPEAK *Many confuse these with process and outcome evaluation which the originator,*
Author *Michael Scriven, did not intend. An example is the glossary of terms in "A*
Comment *Framework for the Development of Competency-based Curricula"...In the exam consequently appears to be prudent to choose the definitions that link formative evaluation to process and summative evaluation to outcome.*

Qualitative vs. Quantitative evaluation

Qualitative evaluation data begin as descriptive information about programs and peop programs whereas, quantitative data can tell us whether change can be attributed to interventio how much change there was in a program. Qualitative data can give us clues about why an intervention worked or did not work. For example, an observer might note that the relationship between the trainer and the trainees seems warmer with more interaction in one group than in a comparison group receiving similar skill training.

Qualitative methods produce large detail on smaller numbers of people and cases and constrained by predetermined categories. Quantitative data uses standardized measures that fit responses into predetermined categories and can measure reactions of many to a limited set of questions. The latter facilitates comparison and statistical aggregation of data and provides a b generalizable set of findings.

Qualitative descriptions of processes are useful in understanding the dynamics of program operations; revealing areas in which programs can be improved, highlighting the strengths of the programs permitting people not closely involved to understand how a program operates. Useful for dissemination and replication of programs under conditions where a program has served as a demonstration project or is considered to be a model worthy of replication at other sites. Highly individualized programs that have individual goals such as tailored health promotion programs or counseling interventions may lend themselves to case descriptions. Validity and reliability are dependent upon trained, structured, consistent observations and reporting.

Qualitative methods consist of three kinds of data collection:
in-depth interviews
direct observations
written documents (including questionnaires, personal diaries, program records)

The purposes and functions of these two methods are different but complementary. They are being used more together as multiple methods of evaluation have been encouraged. Subsequent comments are focused on quantitative evaluation.

Sources of Data for Evaluation
Records, agencies, census and vital statistics; program participants; staff delivering program; family members or significant others; reports, observations of evaluator; community-level indexes

Evaluation Steps
Plan evaluation while program planning and before implementation
a. Choose the evaluation question, define purpose of evaluation–who wants to evaluate? Who are the stakeholders. Identify changes that can (should) be attributed to program
b. Select indicators for success of objectives (See Section II – Planning page 31)
List levels of evaluation (Review Figure 11 page 51)
Plan evaluation–steps (See Stepp Model page 50)
c. Evaluation design (purpose of the design is to eliminate systematic bias) What data need to be collected to answer what question? Select the comparison.
d. Plan data collection; who, when, where, how, by whom, when
e. Identify or design measurement instruments
f. Select test statistics to determine degree and significance of changes detected

Implementation
Management of evaluation–training of collectors, supervise, monitor
Data collection and reduction
•Analysis and interpretation of findings

• Reporting evaluation and advocating for change

The objective of the evaluation is to get the findings utilized by the decision m
and get the results incorporated into planning and implementation or to make
modifications or recommendations.

Concepts

Cost benefit - A measure of the cost of an intervention relative to the benefits
yields, usually expressed as a ratio of dollars saved or gained for every dollar
on the program.

Cost effectiveness - A measure of the cost of an intervention relative to its im
usually expressed in dollars per unit of effect. *(Green 1986)*

Norm referenced - Individual performance is compared to others in group (e
grading on the curve).

Criterion referenced testing - Individual performance viewed as direct meas
content or skill assessed by test, no reference to others.

Ethical standards -

    Treatment of involved people

    Role conflicts

    Scientific quality of evaluation

    Recognizing needs of all stakeholders

    Negative effects

       Inaccurate findings can hurt people

    Type I & Type II errors

    Unplanned program effects

Validity and reliability of instruments: Reliability is the extent to which the instrum
will produce the same score if applied to an object two or more times.

Validity is the extent to which the instrument measures what the evaluator wants it to
measure or claims that it measures.

II EVALUATION DESIGNS

Concepts

Sampling is a process by which a portion of the population is selected. The goal is to
represent the population as closely as possible and minimize bias due to selection.

Probability—sample in which all elements of the population in a universe have a kno
probability of being selected.

Probability sample is important because it is the only type of sample that allows the ev
to treat the sample as technically representative of the larger population. Examples: simple ran
stratified random, cluster samples.

Non-probability samples are not representative. Examples: convenience samples,
homogeneous & heterogeneous samples.

Variable = name for an object of interest that is thought to influence (or be influenced something else. Independent (cause), dependent (effect) variables.

Language of design - 0 = observation X = intervention or experiment R = randomization. Designs are intended to measure change and determine if change is a result of the intervention. Things that can get in the way of the latter are called threats to validity (what can distort the outcome): history, maturation, instrumentation, testing, selection, Hawthorne effect, attrition.

a. Non experimental approaches (single group designs) can assess usefulness of further evaluation; correlate improvements with other variables; prepare facility for further evaluation.

These designs answer: How well are the participants functioning at the end of the program? Are minimum standards of outcome achieved? How much do participants change during their participation in the program? **They will not tell you that change was the result of the intervention/program.**

Single group designs/ Non experimental

One observation X 0

Two observations 0_1 X 0_2 (also called pre/post test)

---

b. Quasi-experimental designs help evaluators identify if changes in program participants were the result of the program. This is done through 1) observing participants at additional times before and after the program, 2) observing additional people who have not received the program, 3) using a variety of variables some expected to be influenced by the program and others not expected to be affected. Particular health education concerns are biases caused by self-selection into program; general community or societal changes; and the reactive effects of making observations.

Quasi-experimental Design Examples

Comparison group without pre-test design	0 X 0
	X 0
Comparison group design	0 X 0
	0 0
Time Series	0 0 0 X 0 0 0 0

The five elements of evaluation design: 1) representative sample of target population; 2) one or more pretests; 3) unexposed group for comparison; 4) random assignment of the samples; 5) one or more post tests to measure effects after the experimental intervention.

True experimental or research design requires random assignment to control for bias and having all the elements that are listed above as the elements of research/evaluation design.

III DATA ANALYSIS

Statistics in education have these purposes:

    a. summarize information such as measures of central tendency and measures dispersion or variability

    b. to determine how seriously to regard differences observed: are they real or chance occurrence

    c. determine the amount of relationship between data sets; correlation (correla an advance over percentages because it allows you to capture in a single statis both the direction and amount of association)

Know four levels of measurement in order to identify meaningful statistical tests

    a. nominal – variables have labels but no inherent meaning
        Example: red apples, yellow apples, green apples
    b. ordinal – implies levels of intensity or severity. One category is
        more or less than another. Categories are in sequence.
        Example: sour apples, tart apples, sweet apples
    c. interval – variables have a standard unit of measure
        e.g. miles; standardized test scores; degrees farenheit
    d. ratio – standard unit of measure with an absolute zero e.g.
        dollars, inches, degrees centigrade

The most frequently occuring category or mode is useful for describing the distribution nominal data. The median is applicable to ordinal level data. The mean is applicable t interval data except where you have extremes or outliers, the median is then used.

Three types of statistics:

    • univariate – distribution, measures of central tendency & dispersion,
        tests of significance
    • bivariate – measures of association - how strong
    • multi-variate – measures of association, tests of signficance,
        variance- measures of dispersion

DEEDSPEAK
Author
Comment

Note: thus far only univariate statistics have been tested for in the exam.

Figure 12
NORMAL
STRIBUTION
OR BELL
CURVE
S FOR TESTS
FICANCE, AS
ELL AS, TEST
GRADING
ROCEDURES

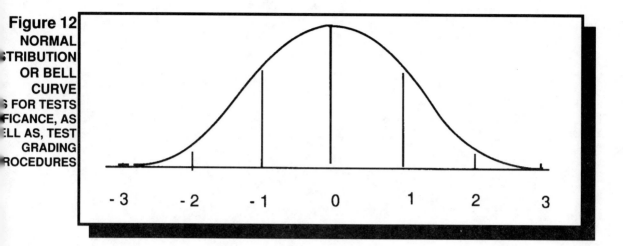

V COORDINATE PROVISION OF HEALTH EDUCATION SERVICES

Key Practice Questions

1. Saying "let the boss or an impartial expert decide" is an example of conflict resolution by: a) compromise; b) problem solving; c) fight or confrontation; d) flight or avoidance.

2. Coalition building is based on: a) an organization's own interests b) collaboration c) representativeness; d) a concern for equity in sharing resources.

3. Leadership, conflict management and goal setting are examples of processes that: a) are not required in the HES role; b) are supplemental concerns in in-service training; c) are equally applicable to team building and to intra-agency collaboration; d) are skills commonly found in every organizational setting.

. H. E. S.

IREMENT

5.1 Elicit the cooperation of persons from diverse programs by establishing relationships with and between those individuals in order to coordinate related health education services

Two major approaches concerning interaction between organizations can be identified: collaboration and negotiation.

A collaborative approach requires organizations to identify unity and agreement between diverse groups, to harmonize ways of working together. A negotiating approach usually is based on different organizations pursuing their own interests. *(Brodie 1982 p. 123).* Collaboration is the basis for coalition building and important early in planning process. It is based on politics, power, and resource allocation.

Conflict management is an important skill in gaining intergroup and intragroup cooperation and collaboration. Conflict to some degree always exists, it is part of life. Therefore the goal is to manage conflict in constructive ways. There are three modes of management. 1. Confrontation/fight includes win-lose power struggles, scapegoating, and third-party judgment. 2. Collaborative confrontation includes problem solving, compromise and peaceful coexistence. 3. Avoidance includes withdrawal, isolation, indifference, and feigned ignorance.

Collaborative problem solving and compromise using negotiation is the most effective strategy. Steps in negotiation: 1) Meet on neutral ground; 2) Actively listen to each other; 3) Assert self responsibly; 4) Lower defenses; 5) Seek consensus; 6) Exercise spirit of compromise; 7) Seek satisfaction on both sides.

It is important to consider the makeup of the organizations when attempting to build collaborative and cooperative relationships.

Human service organizations have three levels or domains: policy , management, and Each approaches problems of service integration differently. Each has its own unique perspec each tends to be in conflict with one or both of the other two domains. Medical Centers are s with three different social systems (board, management, service) as opposed to one in industr systems lead to separate identifiers, interpretations of events, contrasting norms, discordance, for control, different change rhythms, and uncertainty. *(Ross Micco 1980)*

Building interdisciplinary groups or teams as well as interagency collaboration requi dealing with issues such as goal-setting, role expectation, negotiation, decision-making, proble solving, leadership, and conflict management.

Health educators must develop plans for coordination, facilitate cooperation between levels of program personnel and organizations, serve as liaison between groups, employ confli reduction, organize in-service training.

1. Networking - inducing change - power or resource base
   Identify supportive organizational or community
   relationships that benefit programs(s)
   Promote cooperation and feedback
2. Conflict resolution and negotiation skills
3. In-service training
   Functions: identification of effective and efficient strategies and tra
   methods; training of trainers, information and resource gathering, d
   training modules, consultation on training methods, identification o
   and consulting with experts, coordinating training activities, evalua
   design, and implementation of training. *(Standards of Practice 199*

   A. How People Learn *(see also Principles of Learning in Introduc*
   From reading and participating; with emotional impact and in the ₂
   of threat; with illustration, with room for insight; with a framework
   satisfy adult needs, with a sense of responsibility and relevance; in
   comfortable setting and with humor.
   B. Designing Training
   Needs assessment, objectives, use of time & space, preparation,
   evaluation.
   C. Training Methods
   Lecture, large group discussion, small group discussion, audiovisua
   role plays, exercises and games.
   (See also Breckon for more comments on training)
4. Team building

VI ACTING AS RESOURCE PERSON

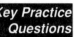

Key Practice Questions

1. Consideration of both individual requester and/or the organization are important when identifying resources to satisfy a health information request. Rank the following factors in order of their priority in fulfilling the request and circle the sequence: A) educational level and occupation; B) reading ability and the subject matter; C) previous experience and cultural background; D) gender and lifestyle. a) ABCD; b) BCAD; c) CABD; d)ADBC.

2. Select the international organization focused on promoting health from the following list: a) WHO; b) UNICEF; c) UNDP; d) World Bank.

3. Identify a voluntary agency from the following list: a) ADA; b) AMA; c) AHA; d) ACS.

4. You have been assigned to write a grant proposal on violent and abusive behavior. Which is the most appropriate data base for initiating your search: a) Psychlit; b) ERIC; c) Medline; d) AIDS Abstracts.

5. If you conduct a data base search for information on harmful levels of certain chemicals in ocean fish consumed in Florida, what combination of key words would provide the best access to the information you need? a) Florida, fish, ocean, eating; b) Fish, chemicals, Florida consumption; c) Florida; pollution, chemicals, fish, consumption; d) Industry, fish, Florida, chemicals.

O rganize and keep up to date: directory of community health information resources; catalog of educational materials; current reference file of resources for health services and community information; a method to access this information by staff and public.

Expand resources: collaborate, recruit volunteers, seek contributions.

. H. E. S.
UIREMENT

6.1 Select sources of information on health issues by evaluating these sources in order to disseminate health information

6.1 UTILIZE HEALTH INFO RETRIEVAL SYSTEMS

Health Data Bases
    Example of key words
    Major electronic data bases: Medline, ERIC, PsychLit, etc.
    Sources for searches

Literature Searches
    Steps: identify need, match needs to likely sources, pursue leads, judge

quantity and quality; organize materials in useful form—categorize reference, catalogue

Standard Sources of Material

Libraries – public and university
Government clearinghouses
Professional & voluntary organizations, journals,
    magazines, newsletters
State departments - health, education
Local sources, organizations, newspapers, reports,

Government Clearinghouses

For lists of clearing houses for health issues write:
National Health Information Clearinghouse
PO Box 1133
Washington, D.C. 20013-1133

6.1 INTERPRET & RESPOND TO HEALTH INFO REQUESTS

Match information with requests; match organizational context and requester, educati cultural, social levels. Select materials (see below), know limitations of information, match re with responders. Be able to systematically organize for requests and needs.

6.1 SELECT EFFECTIVE MATERIALS FOR DISSEMINATION

Use of instructional media – purpose, selection, standards, resources.

Criterion: health information materials must: have planned use; relate to interested au potential consumers or special population groups in terms of age, culture, language, education literacy levels; incorporate principles of good publication design; be technically accurate; be p for accuracy, appropriateness and effectiveness; be actively used and distributed; be kept curre *(Standards of Practice 1991)*

Know and apply community standards – accuracy, community customs and acceptab

Fodor & Dalis criteria check list: contain a core of accurate information; at appropria maturity level; economical in terms of time expended; readily available; expose clients to a va information; enable clients to acquire information at their own pace.

Breckon on effective development of materials: Printed materials should be attractiv interesting, uncluttered, readable, concise, important, timely, clear, motivating, and accurate.

Pretesting – 1. Planning and strategy selection; 2. Concept development; 3. Message execution.

Readability – Using a formula to predict the approximate grade level a person must have achieved in order to understand written material. It is based on the number of polysyllabic words and the length of the sentence. There are a number of readability formulae known by acronyms such as SMOG and FOG.

6.2 Serve as consultant by assisting in the identification of issues and recommending alternative strategies

6.2 CONSULTATIVE RELATIONSHIPS

- **Consultation – Purpose:** establish a helping relationship.
- **Definition:** a consultant is a person who is trying to have some influence over a group or organization but has no direct power to make changes or implement programs. *(Block)*
  Consultation is a two-way interaction — a process of seeking, giving, and receiving help. *(Lippett & Lippett 1978)*
- **Cardinal condition:** help is never really help unless and until it is perceived as helpful by the recipient, regardless of the helper's good intentions.
- Consultation is a conceptual tool for change agent role for individual, interpersonal, organizational, or inter-organization change (other change agent tools are training and research). Different from other roles such as training, supervision, administrative, counselling.
- Characteristics of the relationship: permissive, voluntary, temporary, supportive, disciplined, interactive – two-way process, and initiated by the consultee.
- Two components: technical expertise and an emotional component.
- Models – expert, pair of hands, collaborative or problem solver.
- Six phases of consultation *(Lippett & Lippett 1978)*
     1. Contact and entry
     2. Contract and establish relationship
     3. Problem identification - analysis
     4. Goal setting and planning
     5. Taking action and cycling feedback
     6. Contract completion - design continuity and terminate

VII COMMUNICATION

Key Practice Questions

1. A SMOG test measures: a) impact of a visual image; b) reading level; c) scope of information in a document; d) air quality in Rio.

2. Select the correct statement: a) fear messages in health education are never used because they are ineffective; b) fear messages are effective if they include an action which will reduce the fear; c) fear messages are effective in moderation; d) fear messages are unpopular.

3. Most health educators continuously employ this technique to change behavior: a) persuasive communication; b) advocacy; c) ethical conduct; d) group dynamics.

. H. E. S.
UIREMENT

VII COMMUNICATE HEALTH AND HEALTH EDUCATION NEEDS, CONCERNS, AND RESOURCES

7.1 Keep abreast professional literature, current trends, and research
7.2 Advocate for inclusion of education in health programs and services
7.3 Explain the foundations of the discipline of health education including its purposes, theories, history, ethics, and contributions in order to promote the development and practice of health education

The skill requirements that were used to set the general context for the field in the introduction are restated here as they can also be applied to individual workers and to specific health education activities. The subject matter of health education to be interpreted is derived from the biological and behavioral sciences. The goal of health education centers around the promotion of wellness. Health educators must know how to apply learning and social change theories in relation to health, and select and apply theories and concepts, programs and activities.

Professional values must be clear. The health educators must be alert to discrimination, sensitive to the differences between education and manipulation, and able to employ a range of
. H. E. S. strategies for dealing with controversial health issues.
UIREMENT

7.4 Select communication methods and techniques by matching characteristics of individual target group with methods/techniques and issues in order to assess, plan, implement, and evaluate health education services

7.4 SELECT COMMUNICATIONS METHODS AND TECHNIQUES

Health communications programs can: increase awareness of a health issue, problem solution; affect attitudes to create support for individual or collective action; demonstrate or ill skills; increase demand for health services; remind about or reinforce knowledge, attitudes or behavior.

Health communications programs cannot: compensate for a lack of health care servic produce behavior change without supportive program components; be equally effective in addr all issues or relaying all messages.

Theories and models used in planning health communications programs come from sc marketing, health education, and mass media.

Social marketing = principles and techniques of marketing to increase effectiveness o programs aimed at producing social change. Four P's of marketing: Product, Promotion, Place *(Kotler 1987)* Dever points up relationship of epidemiology and social marketing saying both strengthen the fit between the health services offered and the needs of the populations saying "marketing theory is based on a systemic view of organizations in which their functioning is vi terms of exchange." *(Dever 1991)*

See Appendix I for communications persuasion model page 101.

COMMUNICATIONS SKILLS

1. ORAL - INFORMAL SKILLS Establish rapport, listening skills – read body langua paraphrase, give and get feedback

2. ORAL FORMAL SKILLS Public speaking – organization, delivery, use of audio-vi

3. WRITTEN SKILLS Adequate preparation, audience analysis, tone; composition– clarity, coherence, conciseness, correctness

4. PUBLIC RELATIONS AND MARKETING - PR concerned about images and is a management tool. Marketing is concerned about programs and products and works t determine what people want or need and requires consumer rather than provider orientation. Both require plans and knowledge of media markets, surveying, focus gr testing, publicity and design.
Criterion: health educators should maintain liaison with media representatives to coordinate and assure accurate and timely distribution of information via newspapers radio and other media sources. *(Standards of Practice 1991)*

5. MASS MEDIA Know uses, limitations, timing and scope

See Flora, 1989 for four major uses for mass media in health promotion: educator, promoter, supporter, supplementer.

See Green, 1984 "A Macro Intervention to Support Health Behavior" for synthesis of communication models.

Concepts
•Gatekeepers or Opinion Leaders – Research on the process of personal influence suggests a movement of information through two basic stages:
First from media to relatively well-informed individuals who frequently attend to mass communications; second, from those persons through interpersonal channels to individuals who had less direct exposure to media and who depend upon others for their information — **this is called the two-step flow of communication** and is related to the adoption of innovation concept. (See page 78)

GLOSSARY OF COMMUNICATION TERMS

from "Making Health Communication Programs Work"

Attention. A pretesting measure to describe a message's ability to attract listener or viewer attention; this is often called "recall."

Attitudes. An individual's predispositions toward an object, person or group, which influence his or her response to be either positive or negative, favorable or infavorable, etc.

Baseline study. The collection and analysis of data regarding a target audience or situation prior to intervention.

Central location intercept interviews. Interviews conducted with respondents who are stopped at a highly trafficked location that is frequented by individuals typical of the desired target audience.

Channel. The route of message delivery (e.g., mass media, community, interpersonal).

Closed-ended questions. Questions that provide respondents with a list of possible answers from which to choose; also called multiple choice questions.

Communication concepts. Rough art work and statements that convey the idea for a full message.

Communication strategy statement. A written statement that includes program objectives, target audiences, an understanding of the information needs and perceptions of each target audience, what actions they should take, the reasons why they should act and the benefits to be gained. This document provides the direction and consistency for all program messages and materials.

Comparison group. A control group randomly selected and matched to the target population according to characteristics identified in the study to permit a comparison of changes between those who receive the intervention and those who do not.

Comprehension. A pretesting measure to determine whether messages are clearly understood.

Convenience samples. Samples that consist of respondents who are typical of the target audience and

who are easily access[...] not statistically projec[...] the entire population [...] studied.

Diagnostic informati[...] Results from pretestin[...] research that indicate [...] strengths and weakne[...] in messages and mat[...]

Focus group intervie[...] type of qualitative rese[...] in which an experienc[...] moderator leads abou[...] 10 respondents throug[...] discussion of a selec[...] topic, allowing them t[...] freely and spontaneou[...]

Formative evaluatio[...] Evaluative research conducted during prog[...] development. May inc[...] state-of-the-art review[...] pretesting messages [...] materials, and pilot te[...] program on a small sc[...] before full implementa[...]

Frequency. In adverti[...] used to describe the [...] number of times an a[...] is exposed to a specif[...] media message.

Gatekeeper. Someon[...] must work with before[...] can reach a target au[...] (e.g., a schoolteacher[...] accomplish a task (e.[...] television public servi[...]

director).

Goal. The overall improvement the program will strive to create.

Impact Evaluation. Research designed to identify whether and to what extent a program contributed to accomplishing its stated goals (here, more global than outcome evaluation).

In-depth interviews. A form of qualitative research consisting of intensive interviews to find out how people think and what they feel about a given topic.

Intermediaries. Organizations, such as professional, industrial, civic, social or fraternal groups, that act as channels for distributing program messages and materials to members of the desired target audience.

Objective. A quantifiable statement of a desired program achievement necessary to reach a program goal.

Open-ended questions. Questions that allow an individual to respond freely in his or her own words.

Outcome evaluation. Research designed to account for a program's accomplishments and effectiveness; also called "impact" evaluation.

Over-recruiting. Recruiting more respondents than required to compensate for expected "no-shows."

Polysyllabic words. Words that contain three or more syllables.

Pretesting. A type of formative research that involves systematically gathering target audience reactions to messages and materials before they are produced in final form.

Probe. Interviewer techniques used to solicit additional information about a question or issue. Probe should be neutral (e.g., "What else can you tell me about _____?") not directive ("Do you think the pamphlet was suggesting that you take a particular step-such as changing your diet?")

Process evaluation. Evaluation to study the components of program implementation; includes assessments of whether materials are being distributed to the right people and in what quantities, whether and to what extent program activities are occurring, and what other measures of how and how well the program is working.

PSA. Public service announcement, used without charge by the media.

HEALTH EDUCATION IN SCHOOL SETTINGS

1. For an epidemic of absenteeism in the school which data source would you use first to identify a health education intervention? a) daily attendance records; b) phone calls to parents; c) interviews with students; d) physician medical records.

2. Which group is most influential in planning school health education content? a) teachers; b) parents; c) doctors; d) school nurses.

3. Which group is most influential in implementing health education content? a) teachers; b) parents; c) doctors; d) school nurses.

4. You are planning a health education curriculum for schools. What's the least important consideration? a) individual teacher comments; b) administrator perspectives; c) textbooks; d) parental attitudes.

5. You are assigned to develop a teen-age pregnancy reduction program in a high school. The objective is to reduce the number of unwanted pregnancies within five years. The best theoretical base for planning behavior changes to give you a wide range of interventions is: a) health belief model; b) social learning theory; c) the adoption-diffusion model; d) stages of change.

6. In the above example, the important target for your planned training in skill and attitude change will be: a) administrators; b) volunteers; c) school nurses; d) teachers.

7. From the following, identify the component that is not central to the comprehensive school health model: a) healthy school environment; b) a student health parent participation group; c) health education; d) health services.

PURPOSE – Protect, maintain, and promote the health of the children and adults who live and work together every day of the school year. School must maintain health of students to ensure continued fitness to learn; maintain environment that contributes to health; do best to ensure optimum health through appropriate health services; educate children to make sound decisions on health-related matters. Wellness-oriented, comprehensive, sequentially organized health instruction makes a strong, effective program. *(Pollock & Hamburg 1985)*

PROCESSES – The goal is comprehensive school program integrating health instruction, services, and environment. Health teaching must be integrated into all appropriate areas of curriculum. Work with families. Adults in schools provide models for behaviors. Some schools are beginning to provide health promotion programs for staff and teachers. Community practices interact and overlap with schools. The focus is on curriculum development and teaching skills, along with health content.

DEFINITIONS *(Joint Committee on Terminology 1990)*

Comprehensive School Health Program – An organized set of policies, procedures, a[ ]
activities designed to protect and promote the health and well-being of students and staff whic[ ]
traditionally included health services, healthful school environment and health education. It s[ ]
also include, but not be limited to, guidance and counseling, physical education, food service, [ ]
work, psychological services, and employee health promotion.

School Health Education – One component of the comprehensive school health prog[ ]
which includes the development, delivery, and evaluation of a planned instructional program [ ]
other activities for students pre-school through grade 12, for parents and for school staff, and i[ ]
designed to positively influence the health knowledge, attitudes, and skills of individuals.

Comprehensive School Health Instruction – The development, delivery, and evaluati[ ]
planned curriculum, pre-school through 12 with goals, objectives, content sequence, and speci[ ]
classroom lessons which includes, but is not limited to, the following major content areas: [ ]
community health, consumer health, environmental health, family life, mental and emotional [ ]
injury prevention and safety, nutrition, personal health, prevention and control of disease, subs[ ]
use and abuse.

Post-Secondary Health Education Program – A planned set of health education polic[ ]
procedures, activities, and services that are directed to students, faculty and/or staff of college[ ]
universities, and other higher education institutions. This includes, but is not limited to: gene[ ]
health courses for students, employee and student health promotion activities, health services, [ ]
professional preparation of health educators and other professionals, self-help groups, student

---

ASSESSMENT – The target groups for school health is kids, a captive audience. They are m[ ]
healthy, which makes for a positive approach as opposed to a disease or problem focus. The s[ ]
administrators are the decision makers for school health programs. Federal, state, and local po[ ]
and resources influence the status as do community needs and pressures. Interview administrat[ ]
parents, students and teachers when determining curriculum. Needs assessment determines the [ ]
and sequence of the curriculum. Link health-related behavioral problems and solutions to age [ ]
and to cultural groups. Analyze students' health beliefs based on Health Belief Model, Piaget's[ ]
Cognitive Development Theory. Elementary teacher is the critical provider for health instructi[ ]
Tools used: records including student files, cumulative records; interviews with parents, [ ]
administrators, teachers, school nurse; surveys, community data.

PLAN – Equip children with fundamental health concepts and problem-solving skills that will [ ]
sound decision-making in the future. State and local health & safety codes must be considered[ ]

School policies impact health instruction. The sources of school health education curriculum are based on answers to basic questions such as "What goals, what changes, what personal developments are of most worth, and what curriculum plans are most likely to achieve them?" *(Pollock & Hamburg 1985)*

IMPLEMENT – Classroom teachers deliver the health education in elementary schools. Some health-trained teachers in junior and senior high school. School nurses are critical. Curriculum development and instructional skills and small group discussion skills are major needs in classrooms.

EVALUATE – needs which help determine the scope and emphasis of health instruction, assess strengths and weaknesses of program (process) and assess extent to which desired outcomes are attained (impact). Emphasis on pre/post tests. Use evaluation data formatively as basis for revisions in course methodology. Few school programs are able to follow-up and assess long-range outcomes, except for specially funded programs. Many in school health believe that teachers and schools can only be held accountable for students' health knowledge and skills.

COORDINATE – Identify, organize and coordinate school and community resources utilized in health instruction program. Synchronize with voluntary agencies and community health campaigns to multiply effect.

RESOURCES – Select community resources not in conflict with school point of view. Select resources suitable to maturity level of learner. Choose materials that contain valid health content and concepts. Identify school and community resources that can enrich health instruction. Accumulate and organize health materials, contacts, and sources.

COMMUNICATE – Models appreciation of health values and zest for living. Sensitive to needs of learners and health levels of students. Delivers messages that are not too sophisticated or too mundane.

ISSUES – Local control over organized curricula--states prescribe subjects at what grade level but not always for health education. Community control and concern over content. Teaching values and morals is most controversial, particularly around sexuality education. Finding funding for faculty positions in health education, finding time for health instruction, and finding teaching staff that are health specialists are problems of administrators seeking to implement comprehensive school health education programs.

ROLES – Develop and evaluate curricula for health; classroom teacher implements health curriculum developed by others; health educator content specialist and trainer; community health educators serve as subject matter experts, curriculum consultants; resource brokers; coordinators and role models.

For universities and colleges, and professional organizations roles are: instructor; consultant, evaluator, student health organizer, coordinator, disseminator of information.

HEALTH EDUCATION SETTINGS

HEALTH EDUCATION IN COMMUNITY SETTINGS

Key Practice Questions

1. You are a consultant in a voluntary organization and see some unethical behavior among employees. Who do you notify? a) the executive director; b) your consultee; c) the board of directors; d) the direct supervisor of the employee.

2. You are a volunteer in a voluntary organization and you see unethical behavior on the part of another volunteer. What do you do? a) speak directly to the volunteer; b) report to the coordinator of volunteers; c) ignore the behavior; d) report it to the administrator.

3. Most voluntary agencies in the health arena are established and based on: a) a single major health problem; b) the Surgeon General's priorities as stated in The Year 2000 Objectives; c) state legislation; d) service delivery concerns.

4. A major problem among voluntary health agencies in the 90's is: a) setting priorities; b) recruiting volunteers; c) securing government funding; d) social marketing.

5. As the health educator for the American Dental Society, your program includes the following objectives: the participants will adopt positive attitudes toward tooth brushing; the participants will rate daily brushing as a highly important activity; 70% of the participants will demonstrate correct use of a toothbrush. These are: a) behavioral objectives; b) process objectives; c) outcome objectives; d) impact objectives.

6. Select the correct response. Evaluation of the objectives above will answer one of the following evaluation questions: a) is our program more effective than a dental care videotape; b) did the health education program make a difference in the dental health of the target group; c) are we using our educational resources as effectively as we can; d) is flossing as important to dental health as brushing daily.

7. The adoption curve illustrates: a) a prediction of the amount of time it takes to get a new idea to an ethnic group; b) that early adopters are healthier and smarter than late adopters; c) the effectiveness of mass media; d) successive waves of adoption by groups with identifiable characteristics.

8. In the social action model of community organization the perception of the constituency group in the community is that they are: a) citizens who can use self-help methods; b) consumers who need facts; c) residents who are victims of the system; d) early adopters.

PURPOSE – to reduce the incidence of health problems or to improve the health status of the community including improving access, changing policies and legislation, shifting community norms. as well as affecting specific behaviors.

Encouraging public participation is more than requesting input; it allows public access
decision-making process, seeks community solutions for institutionalized change, and achieves
partnerships by sharing resources and decision-making power. *(Standards of Practice 1991)*

Definition: *(Joint Committee on Terminology 1990)*

Community Health Education is the application of a variety of methods that result in
education and mobilization of community members in actions for resolving health issues and p
which affect the community. These methods include, but are not limited to, group process, ma
media, communication, community organization, organization development, strategic planning
training, legislation, policy making, and advocacy.

Bracht identifies themes about the process of community-based social and behavioral
(1) Powerful social forces influence individual behavior; behavior formed and influenced by th
dominant culture shapes individual behavior symbolically and tangibly and transmits values an
norms. (2) Communities can be mobilized as a change agent to achieve social and behavioral
Each community is unique but processes to be followed in analysis, design, organization,
implementation, and diffusion of programs are similar. (3) Early and sustained participation b
community members and leaders is necessary for realization of community ownership and pro
maintenance. *(Bracht 1990)*

Green distinguishes between community interventions that seek small but pervasive c
that apply to the majority of the population on a community-wide approach and interventions i
community which seek more intensive or profound change in a sub population, such as a schoc
workplace. The differences are the comparative magnitude of the task and the number of organ
and levels of organization involved. *(Green 1991)*

Community organization: Outcomes are: independent entities working for a mutual g
promotion of cooperation rather than competition among groups; coordination of existing reso
shared leadership, talent, and responsibilities; collaboration and negotiation; community input
decision-making. *(Standards of Practice 1991)*

Three models of community practice *(Ross 1974)*

Community Development – change through broad community participation and con
to develop community capacity, integration, and self-help for economic and social progress. T
clients or targets are the citizens and the power structure are collaborators. Health educator ro
catalyst/coordinator.

Social Planning – change through technical process of problem-solving (use consens
conflict). Rational, controlled change central. Use experts and data, clients are seen as consun
power structure are employers and sponsors. Health educator as fact gatherer, analyst, facilitat

Social Action – organization of disadvantaged segment perhaps with alliances to mak
demands on larger community for resources or justice (conflict model). Aims to redistribute p
resources, basic policies of formal organizations. Clients perceived as victims. Health educator

partisan activist, agitator, negotiator.

PROCESSES – Increased community competence or problem-solving ability is a defining characteristic of a community organization process. *(Ross 1974)* Principle of participation critical at assessment and planning, not just in implementation of programs at this level. Principle of relevance - "starting where people are." Processes of collaboration (when one or more organizations perceive that their own goals can be achieved most effectively and efficiently with the assistance and the resources of others) and negotiation (organization holds discussions with those who evidence varying degrees of resistance to the redistribution of power or resources in the hope of ultimately arriving at an agreement).

ASSESSMENT – Coalition building essential; multi-layer assessments, epidemiological, political, economic, sociological & behavioral; use data sources (see Assessment Section) and interpersonal processes.
Tools: influentials and informants (interview key people); surveys, focus groups, records, census, epidemiological data analysis.

PLAN – Sequencing of activities critical, use of multiple intervention strategies both environmental forces and behavioral patterns-mass media, coalition building, training, skill building, use of existing organizations and resources. Anticipate resistance to change.

IMPLEMENT – Partnerships, participation, coalitions, training, technical assistance, small group dynamics. Development of task forces; development of social system support; organizational commitment to an improved social environment. Track and monitor activity development.

EVALUATE – Plan for evaluation at initial planning stage. Evidence that participation goals are being met, that behavior change strategies are working, that efforts are paying off. Short-term results, changes in policies, allocations, community norms, documented and communicated. Long-term effects require access to epidemiological and community records for comparison and/or baseline data. Plan progress reports, disseminate results to those feeling ownership, interest, or who are affected by the problem.

COORDINATE – Coordinate with community agencies if resources are included in plan; with other health campaigns for synergism; major non-health attention-getters in community —holidays, drives, campaigns, etc.

RESOURCES – See Processes above on negotiation and collaboration.

COMMUNICATE – Plan for dissemination of information, creation of climate, adoption of innovation through mass media, minor media, small groups, organizations.

ISSUES – Size of program, politics, power, collaboration.

DEFINITIONS: Participation/involvement- a process in which individuals or communitie identify with a movement and take responsibility jointly with health professionals and others concerned, for making decisions and planning and carrying out activities. *(WHO 1983)*. Comm organization "a health education process or method in which the combined efforts of individua groups, and organizations are designed to generate, mobilize, coordinate, utilize, and/or redistr resources to meet unsolved or emergent health needs or problems."*(Ross 1967)*

ROLES – Health Departments: enforcement and education components as communications specialists - planning interventions that combine community organization, organizational development, group process, communication; advocacy for policies and legislation, work with variety of departments and specialties such as, nurses, environmentalists.
State and Federal: work with other agencies as constituents, grant writing and monitoring communications. Resource development and training.
Voluntary agencies: professional education, public education, supervision and training of vol resource development, materials development.

**Figure 13
THE
CUMULATIVE
ADOPTION
CURVE**
(Rogers 1983)

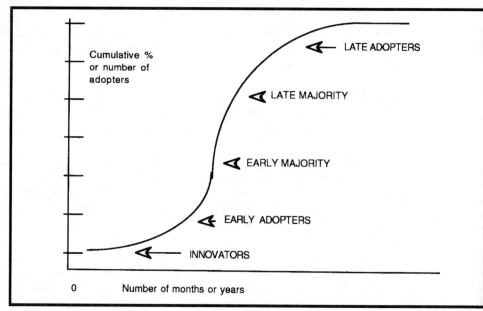

Cumulative %
or number of
adopters

LATE ADOPTERS

LATE MAJORITY

EARLY MAJORITY

EARLY ADOPTERS

INNOVATORS

0   Number of months or years

DESCRIPTION OF ADOPTERS
INNOVATORS   VENTURESOME
EARLY ADOPTERS   RESPECTABLE
EARLY MAJORITY   DELIBERATE
LATE MAJORITY   SKEPTICAL
LAGGARDS   TRADITIONAL

HEALTH EDUCATION IN WORKSITE/OCCUPATIONAL SETTINGS

Key Practice Questions

1. Health Risk Assessment (HRA) data are used in the aggregate to: a) set health insurance rates; b) counsel employees on lifestyle change; c) determine health promotion cost effectiveness; d) plan programs specific to a workplace.

2. HRA data questionnaires can be used individually to: a) set health insurance rates; b) counsel employees on lifestyle change; c) determine health promotion cost effectiveness; d) plan programs specific to a workplace.

3. How can you tell that employees are interested in a smoking cessation program? a) the number who smoke according to a survey; b) attendance at an orientation meeting for smoking classes; c) response to an employer's interview; d) votes at a health promotion planning committee.

4. Absenteeism and alcoholism have been identified as the major problems in a corporation assessment. If you were planning an intervention, what would you select to reduce the absenteeism problem? a) a crisis intervention program; b) a smoking cessation program; c) a stress management program; d) an employee assistance program.

5. What is the health education specialists primary role in wellness programs? a) implementer; b) program planner; c) coordinator; d) technical assistant.

PURPOSE – Specifically, raise morale, reduce absenteeism, reduce unintentional injury or utilization of health care. Also, enhance productivity of workers, reduce employer medical costs— bottom line-enhance profitability. (Business is a major purchaser of health care through worker/retiree health insurance.)

PROCESSES – Relevance, quality, accessibility, and affordability are key concerns; participation of workers and union with management critical in planning and implementing. Organizational assessment of corporate culture important. Internal marketing critical. Must enlist support of upper management.

ASSESSMENT – Health Risk Assessment/Appraisal useful. (See page 21)
Also assess policies, structures, type of industry that create constraints. Medical professionals maintain records that can be used to identify health needs of workers. Employers and unions important to include. Health promotion priorities generally are: reduce smoking, reduce alcohol and drug misuse, improve diet and nutrition, increase physical fitness and exercise, manage stress and violence, in that order. Occupational safety issues are generally not perceived as health education turf.

PLAN – Fit into existing company structure. Target's vary – workers, dependents, retirees. Comprehensiveness is variable. Time allotted – clock time or worker time. Facilities vary. In-community resource use. Consider incentives, competitions, rewards.

IMPLEMENT – Need advisory groups for feedback and adaptation. Continuous communicat results to participants and management. Ways to ration scarce resources: wait list or screen participants, self-help referral to community resources; stepped programs of intervention.

EVALUATE – Plan for evaluation at planning stage. Evidence that participation goals are bei that behavior change strategies are working, that investments are paying off. Short-term result: quantified and communicated. Long-term effects require access to personnel, medical, or insu records for comparison. Plan progress reports, disseminate results.

COORDINATE – Internal departmental coordination needed. Yearly company calendar must coordinate with activities. Coordinate with community agencies if resources are included in pl:

RESOURCES – Total company support to worker supported activities.

COMMUNICATE – Critical to have marketing plan at initiation, continuous monitoring and reporting to management and to workers plus motivational materials.

ETHICAL ISSUES – Confidentiality of records, conflicting loyalties, behavior change vs. environmental/hazard change; labeling and coercion of individuals "victim blaming;" overly-optimistic, misrepresentation of benefits to be derived; unintentional consequences such as discrimination in hiring, compromising medical care benefits. Discrimination against older wo because they use more health care.

ISSUES – Cost benefit data are critical. Start with pilot program to demonstrate effectiveness tactic. Participation of workers a major problem. Focus on worker behavior rather than enviro stresses and hazards problematic. Should focus on both for best program.

ROLES – Plan, implement, evaluate programs; disseminate materials, market to generate management and participant support; facilitate group process and educational assessment skill: budget, evaluation, quality assurance.

Implementor of specific components: adult education skills, motivational skills, mate: development, reporting and recording, as well as content speciality.

HEALTH EDUCATION IN MEDICAL-CARE SETTINGS

Key Practice Questions

1. Your hospital has contracted with the state health department to provide health services to a rural community. A group of new immigrants in the community have an outbreak of measles among their children. They resist immunization. Your job is to develop an education and recruitment campaign quickly to forestall a serious epidemic. You have been unable to develop relationships with this target group beyond minimal contacts and do not have the time to build trust by systematic increments. From the following, select the best alternative step for needs assessment: a) develop a data base of epidemiologic and other records; b) relate to and enlist groups that work with the target group; c) define the problem and action and enlist a spokesperson to translate and relate to the group; d) call the state health department for advice.

2. Assuming that you have been successful in developing a coherent plan to reach out to this group, in what order should the following stakeholders be contacted? A) State health department; B) Local physicians; C) Local newspapers and TV; D) Your hospital administration. Pick the best sequence: a) ABDC; b) BDAC; c) CDAB; d) DABC.

3. Select the behavioral objective for a community program from the following list: a) by 1995 the rate of controlled blood pressure among diagnosed adult hypertensives enrolled in the Lemming Health Maintenance Organization will reach 85%; b) specific lifestyle changes related to non-pharmacologic interventions will be adopted and maintained by 1000 diagnosed hypertensives in the LHMO; c) upon completion of the Total Health Workshop, 80% of the participants will sign a contract to select a lifestyle change; d) participants in the TH workshop will be able to recite a list of 12 fat-free foods.

4. You are the health educator for the hospital clinic that generated the data shown on the clinical cases graph below, representing 113 women. How would you respond to the immediate demand for a priority educational program by the head of the clinic? a) Assure him that you will put it in the budget request for next year; b) gather data to identify the existence of a behavioral component in the problem; c) secure epidemiological and target group data to find out whether this is an episodic chance occurrence or a new trend; d) ask your supervisor for advice.

5. The same graph also indicates infections among a cohort of women and shows the monthly number of new cases of an asymptomatic infection diagnosed and the cumulative number of cases at the end of 6 months. Pick the correct statement from the following: a) the incidence is higher every month; b) the prevalence is variable at every month; c) the prevalence has risen steadily each month; d) the infectious cases identified show that they have been cured within ten days of diagnosis.

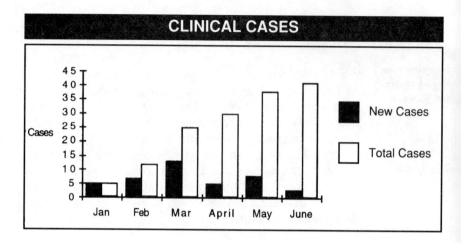

CLINICAL CASES

PURPOSE – Medical care systems are concerned with patient care outcomes, cost effective programs, and community image. Prepaid plans, including HMO's, are concerned with ov utilization. The purpose of patient education is to maintain or improve health, prevent illness c some cases, to slow the deterioration of patients or to educate health professionals to assist thei patients to develop appropriate behaviors. In some cases it is to achieve policies, structures, re allocations in medical care settings to aid reduction of patient morbidity and mortality, increase independence and quality of life. Health promotion and wellness activities are mainly promotic resemble the characteristics of worksite health education.

PROCESSES – Focus mainly on identifiable groups and individuals who have entered the me care system. Health educator identifies philosophical and organizational barriers that hinder or facilitate health education. Works with medical personnel who have contacts with patients.

ASSESSMENT – Hospital and clinic records (utilization, discharge data, readmissions) patien provider surveys, community surveys, marketing surveys are data sources. Concerns of medica personnel important.
Tools: interested party analysis (interview key people); questionnaire checklist, focus groups, structured interviews, community data, tracking patient through system or conducting a system analysis.

PLAN – List all behaviors affecting the particular solution and determine whether policy, struc organizational constraints or specific programmatic approaches will influence provider or patie behavior. Determine which behaviors are most important in affecting health status; determine v behaviors are the easiest to change, given a limited amount of educational time. Focus on skill development, not just on knowledge of disease at patient level. Family and peer support import new patient behaviors.

METHODS – Use national media and local media to develop climate for change if programs are available, computer based education for specific health problems, films/video tapes, brainstorming, role playing, rehearsal, questioning, self monitoring, contracting. One-to-one education most common type, has four major considerations: time available, knowing what to teach, knowing how to teach, and documenting what has been taught. Redmon identifies major differences between learning models used in schools vs. patient education; the goals of cognitive skill and discipline-orientation in school is replaced in patient education by teaching independent problem-solving in an irregular time frame. *(Redmon, 1981)* No single channel of education is inherently superior to another, and the effectiveness of specific interventions depends on their appropriate selection and application. *(Mullen 1990)*

IMPLEMENT – Documentation, tracking and monitoring legal requirement for accreditation. Alternative to patient record is patient check off list. Training for providers continuous.

EVALUATE – Effectiveness measures depend on level of planning, ranges from morbidity and mortality at institution level, to improved utilization, compliance, health status at program level, to specific skills, attitudes, behaviors at patient level.

COORDINATE – Must coordinate delivery of programs with inflexible demands and time tables of medical institutions.

RESOURCES – Community, voluntary agency, and commercial resources can be found for educational materials and services. Be sure to pretest materials and check on most current information.

COMMUNICATE – Patient recruitment depends on marketing to the health professionals and encouraging referrals. Marketing to public depends on making program attractive, affordable, right time, and accessible.

ETHICS – Atmosphere of medical institution intimidating and coercive to patients, difficult to encourage self-management and self-determination.

ISSUES – Adherence or compliance to prescribed regimen, drug interactions, physician-patient interactions. Three strategies to increase adherence to regimen: Correct patients' misconceptions about the regimen, adjust the intervention to patients' lifestyles; enhance support from family members. *(Improving Adherence Among Hypertensive Patients 1987)* The role of the health education specialist vs. provider of service is based on role identification and role responsibilities – health education overall planning, implementation and evaluation of education programs, provider usually one-to-one counseling.

ROLES – Development of community awareness, patient support networks, professional education initiatives. As directors, managers, coordinators of programs focus is often administrative and

supportive rather than educational. As education specialists, curriculum developer, plan, imple
and evaluate programs, select methods and materials and be a staff trainer. As program manage
coordinate teaching assignments and materials, carry out needs assessments and program evalu
budget, report, plan staff development, employee wellness and worksite health promotion.

REFERENCES FOR INTRODUCTION

Baelz, P.R. "Philosophy of Health Education." In Health Education: Perspectives and Choices. Ed. I. Sutherland. London: Allen & Unwin, 1979.

Califano, J. Speech given before the National School Health Conference. Minneapolis, 1977.

Cleary, H.P., J.M. Kichen, and P.G. Ensor. Advancing Health Through Education. Mountain View, Ca.: Mayfield, 1985. A comparison of principles of learning and social change and their application to health education. Page 8 - 9 is useful in connection with principles of learning, page 13.

Faden, R.R. and A.I. Faden. "The Ethics of Health Education as Public Health Policy." HE Monographs (Summer 1985).

Green, L.W. "Determining the Impact and Effectiveness of Health Education as It Relates to Federal Policy." HE Monographs (Supplement, 1978).

Health, United States, and Prevention Profile, 1989. DHHS Pub. No. (PHS) 90-1232. Hyattsville, Md.: National Center for Health Statistics, 1990.

Minkler, M. "Ethical Issues in Community Organization." HE Monographs 6 (Summer 1978).

Pickett, G., and J. Hanlon. Public Health: Administration and Practice. St. Louis: Times Mirror/Mosby, 1990.

Pollock, M.B., and M.V. Hamburg. "Health Education: The Basic of the Basics." In Why School Health Education? The Delbert Oberteuffer Centennial Symposium, AAHE, USDHHS ODPHP, 1985.

Shumaker, S.A., S. Parker, and J. Wolle, eds. The Handbook of Health Behavior Change. New York: Springer, 1990.

REFERENCES FOR NEEDS ASSESSMENT

Breitose, P. Focus Groups–When and how to use them: A Practical Guide. Palo Alto, Ca.: Health Promotion Resource Center, Stanford Center for Research in Disease Prevention, Stanford U School of Medicine, 1988.

Conducting a Community Resource Inventory. Palo Alto Ca.: Health Promotion Resource Center, Stanford Center for Research in Disease Prevention .

Delbecq, A.L. "The nominal group as a technique for understanding the qualitative dimensions of client needs." In Assessing Health and Human Service Needs. Ed. R.A. Bell, et al, 210-218. New York: Human Sciences Press, 1983.

Dever, G.E.A. Community Health Analysis: Global Awareness at the Local Level. Gaithersburg, Md.: Aspen, 1991.

Dignan, M.B., and P.A. Carr. Program Planning for Health Education and Health Promotion. Philadelphia: Lea & Febinger, 1987.

Dillman, D.A. Mail and Telephone Surveys: The Total Design Method. New York: J Wiley & Inc., 1978.

Gilmore, G.D., M.D. Campbell, and B.L. Becker. Needs Assessment Strategies For Health Education and Health Promotion. Indianapolis: Benchmark, 1989.

Gordon, N. So You're Thinking About Conducting A Survey... Oakland, Ca.: Kaiser Permanente, Div. of Research, 3451 Piedmont Ave., 6th Floor, 1990.

Lauffer, A. Assessment Tools. Beverly Hills, Ca.: Sage, 1982.

II REFERENCES FOR PLANNING

Breckon, D., J. Harvey, and R.B. Lancaster. Community Health Education: Settings, Roles & Skills. 2nd ed. Rockville: Aspen, 1989.

Craig, D.P. Hip Pocket Guide to Planning & Evaluation. San Diego: University Associates, Inc., 1978.

DeFries, G., ed. Baseline: A Newsletter of Information About the Evaluation of Health Promotion Programs. Vol. 1:5. Chapel Hill, N.C.: U.N.C., November, 1983.

Dever, G.E.A. Community Health Analysis: Global Awareness at the Local Level. Gaithersburg, Md.: Aspen, 1991.

Green, L.W., and M.W. Kreuter. Health Promotion Planning: An Educational and Environmental Approach. Mountain View, Ca.: Mayfield, 1991.

Green, L.W., M.W. Kreuter, S.G. Deeds, and K.B. Partridge. Health Education Planning: A Diagnostic Approach. Palo Alto, Ca.: Mayfield, 1980.

Rogers, E. Diffusion of Innovations. New York: Free Press, 1983.

Ross, M.G., and B.W. Lappin. Community Organization: Theory, Principles and Practice. 2nd ed. New York: Harper Row, 1967.

Standards of Practice for Public Health Education in California Local Health Departments. CCLDHE, c/o E. Gordon, Ventura Co. PHS, 3161 Loma Vista Rd., Ventura Ca., 93003, 1991.

Sullivan, D. "Model for Comprehensive, Systematic Program Development in Health Education." Health Education 1, no. 1 (Nov-Dec 1973).

Windsor, R.A.; T. Baranowski, N. Clark, and G. Cutter. Evaluation of Health Promotion and Education Programs. Palo Alto, Ca.: Mayfield, 1981.

III REFERENCES FOR IMPLEMENTATION

Forouzesh, M. *Unpublished notes.* CSULB, Long Beach, Ca., 1990.

IV REFERENCES FOR EVALUATION

Craig, D.P. Hip Pocket Guide to Planning & Evaluation. San Diego, Ca.: University Associates, 1978.

Green L.W., and F.M. Lewis. Measurement and Evaluation in Health Education and Health Promotion. Mountain View Ca.: Mayfield, 1986.

Handbook for Evaluating Drug and Alcohol Prevention Programs. USDHHS PHS Pub. No. (ADM) 887: 1512. Washington, D.C.: GPO.

Hoover, K.R. The Elements of Social Scientific Thinking. 4th ed. New York: St. Martin's Press, 1988.

Posevac, E.M., and R.G. Carey. Program Evaluation: Methods and Studies. 3rd ed. Englewood Cliffs, N.J.: Prentice Hall, 1989.

Windsor, R.A., T. Baranowski, N. Clark, and G. Cutter. Evaluation of Health Promotion and Education Programs. Palo Alto, Ca.: Mayfield, 1981.

Program Evaluation Kit. 2nd ed. Newbury Park, Ca.: Sage Pub., 1987. This edition contains nine

books to guide and assist practitioners in planning and managing evaluation. The volumes may
purchased separately or in sets.

V REFERENCES FOR COORDINATION

Beresford, T. How to Be a Trainer. Baltimore: Planned Parenthood of Maryland, 1980.

Breckon, D., J. Harvey, and R.B. Lancaster. Community Health Education: Settings, Roles, &
2nd ed. Rockville, Md.: Aspen Systems, 1989.

Brodie, R. Problem Solving: Concepts and Methods for Community Organizations. New York
Human Sciences Press, 1982.

Building and Maintaining Effective Coalitions. Palo Alto Ca.: Health Promotion Resource Cer
Stanford Center for Research in Disease Prevention, 1990.

Rubin, I.M., M.S. Plovnick, and R.E. Fry. Improving the Coordination of Care: A Program for
Team Development. Cambridge, Mass.: Ballinger, 1975.

VI REFERENCES FOR ACTING AS A RESOURCE PERSON

Block, P. Flawless Consulting: A Guide to Getting Your Expertise Used. Austin, Tx.: Learnin
Concepts, 1981. (Distributed by University Associates, San Diego, Ca.)

Breckon, D.J., J.R. Harvey, and R.B. Lancaster. Community Health Education: Settings, Role:
Skills. 2nd ed. Rockville, Md.: Aspen, 1989.

Fodor, J.T., and G.T. Dalis. Health Instruction: Theory and Application. 4th ed. Philadelphia.
Febiger, 1989.

Lippitt, G., and R. Lippitt. The Consulting Process in Action. San Diego: University Associat
1978.

Schein, E.H. Process Consultation: It's Role in Organization Development.
Addison-Wesley, 1969.

VII REFERENCES FOR COMMUNICATION

Kotler, P., and A.R. Andreasen. <u>Strategic Marketing for Nonprofit Organizations.</u> 3rd ed. Englewood Cliffs, N.J.: Prentice Hall, 1987.

<u>Making Health Communication Programs Work.</u> USDHHS OCC NCI, NIH Pub. No. 89-1493. Washington, D.C.: GPO, April 1989.

McGuire, W. "Theoretical Foundations of Campaigns." In <u>Public Communications Campaigns.</u> Ed. Rice & Paisley. Newbury Park, Ca.: Sage,1981.

REFERENCES FOR SCHOOL SETTINGS

Allensworth, D.D., and C.A. Wolford. "Schools as Agents for Achieving the 1990 Health Objectives for the Nation." <u>Health Education Quarterly,</u> 15 (Spring 1988), 3-15.

DeFriese, G.H., C.L. Crossland, C.E. Pearson, and C.J. Sullivan, eds. "Comprehensive School Health Programs: Current Status and Future Prospects." <u>Journal of School Health,</u> 4 (1990), 127-90.

Fodor, J.T.,and G.T. Dalis. <u>Health Instruction: Theory and Application.</u> 4th ed. Philadelphia: Lea & Febiger, 1989.

Pollock, M.B.,and M.V. Hamburg. "Health Education: The Basic of the Basics." In <u>Why School Health Education?</u> The Delbert Oberteuffer Centennial Symposium, AAHE, USDHHS ODPHP, 1985.

Pollock, M.B.,and K. Middleton. <u>Elementary School Health Instruction.</u> St. Louis: Times Mirror/Mosby, 1989.

"Report of the 1990 Joint Committee on Health Education Terminology." <u>Journal of Health Education</u> 22, no. 2 (March/April 1991).

REFERENCES FOR COMMUNITY SETTINGS

Bracht, N. <u>Health Promotion at the Community Level.</u> Newbury Park, Ca.: Sage, 1990.

Brody, R. <u>Problem Solving, Concepts and Methods for Community Organization.</u> New York: Human Sciences Press, Inc., 1982.

Deeds, S.G., and S. Gunatilake. "Behavioral Change Strategies to Enhance Child Survival." <u>Hygie</u> 8, no. 4 (1989).

Flora, J.A., E.W. Maibach, and N. Maccoby. "The Role of Media Across Four Levels of Health Promotion Intervention." American Review of Public Health 10 (1989): 181-201.

Green, L.W., and A. McAlister. "Macro-Intervention to Support Health Behavior: Some Theor Perspectives and Practical Reflections." Health Education Quarterly 2, no. 3. (1984): 323-339

Hersey, J.C., L.S. Klibanoff, D.J. Lam, and R.I. Taylor. "Promoting Social Support: The Impa California's 'Friends Can be Good Medicine' Campaign." Health Education Quarterly 11 (1984 311.

Lau, R., R. Kane, S. Berry, et al. "Channeling Health: A Review of the the Evaluation of Telev Health Campaigns." Health Education Quarterly 7 (1980): 56-89.

Rothman, J. "Three Models of Community Organization Practice." In Strategies of Communi Organization. F.M. Cox. 2nd ed. Itasca, Ill.: Peacock Pub., 1974.

Schiller, P., A. Steckler, L. Dawson, and F. Patton. Participatory Planning in Community Heal Education: A Guide Based on the McDowell County, West Virginia Experience. Oakland, Ca. Party, 1987.

"World Health Organization: New Approaches to Health Education in Primary Health Care." Technical Report Series 690 (1983): 14.

REFERENCES FOR WORKPLACE SETTINGS

Bertera, R.L. "Planning and Implementing Health Promotion in the Workplace: A Case Study Du Pont Company Experience." Health Education Quarterly 17 (Fall 1990): 307-327.

Parkinson, R.S., et al. Managing Health Promotion in the Workplace: Guidelines for Impleme and Evaluation. Palo Alto Ca.: Mayfield, 1982.

Sloan, R.P. "Workplace Health Promotion: A Commentary on the Evolution of a Paradigm." Education Quarterly 14, no. 2 (Summer 1987): 181-194.

Warner, K.E., T.M. Wickizer, R.A. Wolfe, et al. "Economic Implications of Workplace Health Promotion Programs: Review of the Literature." Jounal of Occupational Medicine 30 (1988): 112.

REFERENCES FOR MEDICAL CARE SETTINGS

Deeds, S.G., B.J. Hebert, and J.M. Wolle. A Model for Patient Education Programming. Washington, D.C.: American Public Health Association, 1979.

Green, L.W., P.D. Mullen, and R.B. Friedman. "Epidemiological and Community Approaches to Patient Compliance." In Patient Compliance in Medical Practice and Clinical Trials. Eds. Cramer and Spilker. New York: Raven Press, 1991.

Improving Adherence Among Hypertensive Patients: The Physician's Guide. USDHHS PHS NIH, March 1987.

Janz, N.K., and M.H. Becker. "The Health Belief Model: A Decade Later." Health Education Quarterly 11 (1984): 1-47.

Mullen, P.D., and L.W. Green. "Educating and Counseling for Prevention: From Theory and Research to Principles." In Preventing Disease: Beyond the Rhetoric. Eds. Goldbloom & Lawrence. New York: Springer-Verlag, 1990.

Redman, B.K. Patterns for Distribution of Patient Education. New York: Appleton-Century-Crofts, 1981.

Rosenstock, I.M., V.J. Strecher, and M.H. Becker. "Social Learning Theory and the Health Belief Model." Health Education Quarterly 15, no. 2 (Summer, 1988): 175-183.

Squyres, W.D. Patient Education: An Inquiry into the State of the Art. New York: Springer, 1980.

Zapka, J., and J.A. Mamon. "Integration of Theory, Practitioner Standards, Literature Findings, and Baseline Data: A Case Study in Planning Breast Self-examination Education." Health Education Quarterly 9 (1982): 332-56.

REFERENCES FOR THEORIES AND MODELS OF BEHAVIOR CHAN

Glaser, B.G., and A.L. Strauss. <u>The Discovery of Grounded Theory: Strategies for Qualitative</u> <u>Research.</u> Chicago: Aldine-Atherton, 1967.

Green, L.W., and M.W. Kreuter. <u>Health Promotion Planning: An Educational and Environme</u> <u>Approach.</u> 2nd ed. Mountain View, Ca.: Mayfield, 1991.

Green, L.W., M.W. Kreuter, S.G. Deeds, and K.B. Partridge. <u>Health Education Planning: A</u> <u>Diagnostic Approach.</u> Mountain View Ca.: Mayfield, 1980.

Lewin, K. "Field Theory in Social Science." <u>Selected Theoretical Papers.</u> Ed. D. Cartwright. York: Harper & Row, 1951.

Maslow, A.H. <u>Toward a Psychology of Being.</u> 2nd ed. New York: Van Nostrand Reinhold, 1

Mullen, P.D., and R. Reynolds. "The Potential of Grounded Theory for Health Education Rese Linking Theory and Practice." <u>Health Education Monographs</u> 6, no. 2 (Spring 1978): 280-29

INDIVIDUAL CHANGE MODELS

Ajzen, I., and M. Fishbein. <u>Understanding Attitudes and Predicting Social Behavior.</u> Englewc Cliffs, N.J.: Prentice Hall, 1980.

Bandura, A. <u>Social Foundations of Thought and Action: A Social Cognitive Theory.</u> Englewc Cliffs, N.J.: Prentice Hall, 1986.

Bandura, A. <u>Social Learning Theory.</u> Englewood Cliffs, N.J.: Prentice Hall, 1977.

Becker, M.H., and I.M. Rosenstock. "Comparing Social Learning Theory and the Health Beli Model." In <u>Advances in Health Education and Promotion.</u> Vol. 2. Ed. W.B. Ward. Greenwic Press, 1987 (245-249).

Diclemente, C.C., and J.O. Prochaska. "Process and Stages of Self-Change: Coping and Comp in Smoking Behavior Change." In <u>Coping and Substance Use.</u> Eds. Shiffman and Wills. Orla Academic Press, 1985.

Fishbein, M., and I. Ajzen. <u>Belief, Attitude, Intention and Behavior.</u> Reading, Ma: Addison-V 1975.

Gottlieb, B. Social Networks and Social Support. Newbury Park, Ca.: Sage, 1981.

Janz, N.K., and M.H. Becker. "The Health Belief Model: A Decade Later." Health Education Quarterly 11 (1984): 1-47.

Mecca, A.M., N.J. Smelser, and J. Vasconcellos. The Social Importance of Self Esteem. Berkeley, Ca.: University of California Press, 1989.

Minkler, M.M. "Applications of Social Support Theory to Health Education: Implications for Work with Elderly." Health Education Quarterly 8 (1981): 147-165.

Pomerleau O.F., and J.P. Brady. Behavioral Medicine: Theory and Practice. Baltimore, Md.: Williams & Wilkins, 1979.

Rosenstock, I.M., V.J. Stretcher, and M.H. Becker. "Social Learning Theory and the Health Belief Model." Health Education Quarterly 15, no. 2 (1988): 175-183.

Skinner, B.F. About Behaviorism. New York: Knopf, 1974.

Stretcher, V.J., B.M. Devellis, M.H. Becker, and I.M. Rosenstock. "The Role of Self-Efficacy in Achieving Health Behavior Change." Health Education Quarterly 13 (1986): 73-91.

Wallston, K.S., and B.N. Wallston. "Health locus of control." Health Education Monographs 6, no. 2 (Spring 1978): 101-170.

Wallston, K.S., and B.N. Wallston. "Who is responsible for your health? The Construct of Health Locus of Control." In Social Psychology of Health and Illness. Eds. G. Sanders and J. Suls. Hillsdale, N.J.: Lawrence Erlbaum, Assoc., 1982. (65 -95)

COMMUNCATION THEORIES AND MODELS

Defleur, M.L., and S. Ball-Rokeach. Theories of Mass Communication, 1989.

Festinger, L. A Theory of Cognitive Dissonance. Stanford, Ca.: Stanford University Press, 1962.

Green, L.W., and A.L. McAlister. "Macro Intervention to Support Health Behavior: Some Theoretical Perspectives and Practical Reflections." Health Education Quarterly 2, no. 3. (1984): 323-339.

Hovland, C.I., I.L. Janis, and H.H. Kelly. Communications and Persuasion. New Haven, Conn: Yale University Press, 1953.

McGuire, W. "Theoretical Foundations of Public Communications Campaigns." In <u>Public Communications Campaigns.</u> Eds. Rice and Paisley. Newbury Park, Ca.: Sage, 1981, 41-70.

Rank, H. "Teaching About Public Persuasion." In <u>Teaching About Doublespeak.</u> Ed. D. Dietri Urbana, Ill.: National Council of Teachers of English, 1976.

COMMUNITY LEVEL

Berlo, D.K. <u>The Process of Communication.</u> New York: Holt, Rinehart & Winston, 1960.

Rogers, E.S. <u>The Diffusion of Innovation.</u> New York: Free Press, 1983.

Rothman, J. "Three Models of Community Organization Practice." <u>In Strategies of Communic Organization.</u> Ed. F.M. Cos et al. 3rd ed. Peacock, F.E., 1979.

MAJOR JOURNALS FOR HEALTH EDUCATORS

AMERICAN JOURNAL OF HEALTH PROMOTION
1812 S. Rochester Rd., Suite 200
Rochester Hills, MI 48307

AMERICAN JOURNAL OF PREVENTIVE MEDICINE
American College of Preventive Medicine
Oxford University Press
2001 Evans Road
Cary, NC 27513

AMERICAN JOURNAL OF PUBLIC HEALTH
The American Public Health Association
1015 15th St., N.W.
Washington, D.C. 20015

HEALTH EDUCATION
The Association for the Advancement of Health Education
1900 Association Drive
Reston, VA 22091

HEALTH EDUCATION QUARTERLY
Society for Public Health Education
2001 Addison Street, Suite 220
Berkeley, CA 94704

HEALTH VALUES
PNG Publications
P.O. Box 4593
Star City, WV 26504

HYGIE
International Union for Health Education
c/o Institut Sante` et Developpement
15-21, rue de l'Ecole de Medecine
F-75270 Paris Cedex 06 France

JOURNAL OF SCHOOL HEALTH
American School Health Association
P.O. Box 708
Kent, OH 44240

PATIENT COUNSELLING and HEALTH EDUCATION
Excerpta Medica
P.O. Box 3085
Princeton, NJ 08540

HEALTH EDUCATION PROFESSIONAL ORGANIZATIONS

*Association for the Advancement of Health Education (AAHE)

The Association for the Advancement of Health Education is part of the larger American Alliance for Health, Physical Education, Recreation, and Dance, which comprises more than 43,000 professionals in sports, dance, safety education, physical education, recreation, and health education. AAHE has a membership of more than 6,500 professionals from schools, universities, community health agencies, and voluntary agencies. It promotes comprehensive health education programming in schools, colleges, and community settings. AAHE has a full-time staff that maintains close contact with legislative issues in Washington, D.C. For further information contact AAHE, 1900 Association Drive, Reston, Va. 22091. 703-476-3437. Bimonthly journal, Health Education. Quarterly newsletter, HE-Xtra.

* American College Health Association (ACHA)

The American College Health Association is made up of individuals and institutions of higher education dealing with health problems and issues in academic communities. It promotes continuing education, research, and program development related to educational institutions. With the increased amount of health education programming in college and university health services, ACHA has become an important forum for health education functioning in those settings. For additional information, contact ACHA,1300 Picard Drive, Suite 200, Rockville, Md. 20850. 410-859-1500. Bi-monthly journal, Journal of the American College Health Association.

*American Public Health Association (APHA)

The American Public Health Association is the largest and oldest membership public health organization in the United States with 50,000 members. It represents the major disciplines and specialists related to public health from community health planning and dental health to statistics and veterinary public health. APHA has two sections of primary interest to health educators: The Public Health Education & Health Promotion Section and the School Health Education and Services Section.

The Public Health Education and Health Promotion Section has more than 2,000 members and is one of the larger sections of APHA. It is concerned with articulating health education roles and advocating for health education concerns throughout the overall APHA organization and its various sections and state affiliates. It is a major sponsor of scientific papers related to health education during the APHA annual meetings.

The School Health Education and Services Section advocates within the APHA structure for comprehensive school health. Such input includes the traditional areas of health instruction in schools, school health services, and a healthful school environment. This section sponsors major scientific papers on school health during annual meetings of APHA.

For further information contact APHA, 1015 15th Street, N.W., Washington, D.C. 20015. 202-789-5600. Monthly journal, American Journal of Public Health. The monthly newsletter is Today's Health. Both sections send out newsletters.

*American School Health Association (ASHA)

The American School Health Association is the primary professional organization cor with issues related to school-age children. School health services, healthful school environmer comprehensive school health education are key areas of concern. ASHA provides the major fo discussion of school health issues through annual, regional, and local affiliate meetings as well through publications and journals. ASHA provides leadership in professional preparation and standards for school health educators, school nurses, physicians, and dental personnel. For furt information, contact ASHA, P.O. Box 708, Kent, Ohio 44240. 216-678-1601. Journal name: of School Health.

American Society for Healthcare Education and Training (ASHET)

The American Society for Healthcare Education and Training is a membership organi: representing a diversity of healthcare and educational organizations for the purpose of promotii awareness of the educational needs common to all healthcare personnel, continuation of profes development in management, and participation in national health issues. Health educators in m care settings find this organization particularly helpful. It has local chapters in large cities whic present programs for professional development. The organization is linked to the American H Association and can be reached at ASHET, 340 N. Lakeshore Drive, Chicago, Ill. 60611. 312- 6113. The journal: Journal of Healthcare Education and Training. The quarterly newsletter: D

Association of State and Territorial Directors of Public Health Education (ASTDPHE)

The Association of State and Territorial Directors of Public Health Education membe made up of 65 directors of health education for each state and/or territory and Indian Health Se the U.S. The conference is primarily concerned with developing standards of health education programming at the state level. It has been active recently in developing communication mech. on health education between state health departments and the federal government in matters re health education. The conference is an affiliate of the Association of State and Territorial Hea Officials. For further information on ASTDPHE, contact any state department of public health name of their newsletter is: Conference Call.

International Union for Health Education (IUHE)

The International Union for Health Education is an international professional organiz committed to the development of health education around the world and has constituent, institu and individual memberships. The union cooperates closely with the World Health Organizatio the United Nations Educational, Scientific, and Cultural Organization (UNESCO) in a variety international forums. IUHE has four major objectives aimed at improving health through educ including establishing links between organizations and people working in health education in v countries of the world, facilitating world-wide exchanges of information, promoting scientific and improving professional preparation in health education, and promoting the development of informed public opinion. The Union meets every three years for an international conference.

For more information on the Union contact the North American Regional Office/IUHE, P.O. Box 2305, Station "D", Ottawa, Ontario, Canada, K1P5W5. The quarterly journal: <u>Hygie.</u>

*Society for Public Health Education (SOPHE)

Founded in 1950, the Society for Public Health Education has provided a major leadership role in public health education, both nationally and internationally. The society was formed to promote, encourage, and contribute to the advancement of health for all people by encouraging research, standards of professional preparation and practice, and continuing education for community and public health education. SOPHE has local chapters throughout the United States which provide continuing education and job referrals. It has articulated standards for masters level public health educators, an approval process for baccalaureate level academic programs in community health education, and a code of ethics that is widely cited in health literature. For further information, contact SOPHE, 2001 Addison Street, Suite 220, Berkeley, Ca. 94704. The journal: <u>Health Education Quarterly.</u> The quarterly newsletter: <u>SOPHE News and Views.</u>

*Society of State Directors of Health, Physical Education, and Recreation (SSDHPER)

The Society of State Directors of Health, Physical Education, and Recreation membership comprises directors of school health, physical education, and recreation in state agencies. Its goal is to promote comprehensive statewide programs of school health, physical education, recreation, and safety. The society works closely with the American Alliance for Health, Physical Education, Recreation, and Dance and the other members of the Coalition of National Health Education Organizations. For further information, contact any state department of education.

*These organizations are represented on the National Commission for Health Education Credentialing

SUMMARIES OF SELECTED HEALTH EDUCATION THEORIES AND MODELS

Adoption and Diffusion Theory *(Rogers)* – A process where new products or ideas are introduced or "diffused" to the audience. The message will be accepted (or behavior adopted) based on whether the audience perceives it as beneficial, as in accordance with their needs and values, finds it easy or difficult to understand or adopt, can try the behavior, and feels that results of the trial are viewed positively by their peers. People adopt new ideas and changes at different rates. The socio-economic characteristics of groups and their rate of adoption have been classified into innovators, early adopters, early majority, late majority, and late adopters or hard to reach. The time that it takes for this process is called diffusion and can be taken into account when choosing strategies and interventions. See adoption curve under Community Settings. *(See readings for examples: Green et al: Macro-Intervention to Support Health Behavior; Deeds & Gunitalake: Behavioral Change Strategies....)*

Behavioral Intention *(Fishbein)* – The likelihood of the target audience adopting a desired behavior can be predicted by assessing (and subsequently trying to change or influence) their attitudes toward and perceptions of the benefits of the behavior, along with how they think that their peers will view their behavior. An individual's and society's perceived attitudes are an important predecessor to action.

Behavioral Medicine *(Pomerleau)* – Clinical use of techniques derived from behavior therapy and behavior modification for the evaluation, prevention, management or treatment of physical disease or physiological dysfunction. Concepts behavioral epidemiology, learning and conditioning, biofeedback, and self-management.

Behaviorism *(Skinner)* – Concentrates on external, observable conditions in which behavior takes place. Behavior change is response to environment. Administer positive or negative reinforcers (stimulus), patterns of behavior can be established or learned (response). Respondent or operant conditioning is directed toward manipulation of stimuli to evoke reflex behavior. No intervening mental process,use of reinforcement schedules.

Cognitive Development Theory *(Piaget)* – Four major stages of cognitive development are described, each characterized by qualitatively different schemes and all experienced in order: 1) the sensory-motor stage (birth to age 2); 2) preoperational stage (age 2 - 7); 3) concrete operational stage (age 7-11); 4) formal operational stage (age 11 to adulthood). Preoperational children confuse cause and effects of illness, conceive of health and illness as two separate happenings, not ends of the continuum. Lack ability to generalize between similar experiences, reason egocentrically. At concrete operational stage children tend to see health as ability to perform desired activities. Begin to grasp concept of causal sequencing and gradually become future oriented. At formal operational stage children understand linkages between behavior and health outcomes and recognize individual susceptibility in onset of disease. Has implications for designing successful school health educ

Cognitive Dissonance *(Festinger)* – The simultaneous existence within a person of knowledge and beliefs that do not fit together (dissonance) leads the person to take efforts to m them fit better (dissonance reduction). Dissonance can arise as a consequence of decisions, temptation, group interactions, disagreement with others, forced public compliance, etc. Disson can be reduced by obtaining support from people who already believe, or by persuading others they too should believe what the person wants to persuade himself is true.

Coping Theory *(Folkman & Lazarus)* – Defined as "the person's constantly changin cognitive and behavioral efforts to manage specific external and/or internal demands that are ap as taking or exceeding the person's resources." Takes in personal and situational factors. Eigh distinct ways of coping: confronting, distancing, self-control, seeking social support, accepting responsibility, escape-avoidance, problem-solving and positive reappraisal.

Field Theory *(Lewin)* – Human behavior is in a constant state of dynamic equilibrium quasi-stationary equilibrium caused by two sets of forces working against each other within the individual or the situation. Forces toward behavior change, and those resisting the movement. every action there is a reaction. *(See force-field analysis under Assessment Tools for practical application of this theory.)*

Freezing-Unfreezing Theory *(Lewin)* – a) Unfreezing is a state of readiness-for-chan basic attitudes, motivations and behaviors. b) Problem-diagnosis phase – identification of force and against change, and analysis of those forces in terms of how and where changes can be intr c) Goal-setting phase – establish specific goals and direction. d) Person experiments with rang new behaviors possible and practices those found to be the more desirable. e) Refreezing – ne learnings and changes found to be beneficial are assimilated into more permanent framework o behavior. *(See Stages of Change Theory.)*

Health Belief Model *(Rosenstock, Becker)* – Beliefs about perceived seriousness, susceptibility, benefits, and barriers affect person's health behavior. Each has cognitive elemen what might happen —and an affective component – how deeply one cares about the consequen Cues which mobilize beliefs is second component.

Learned Helplessness *(Seligman & Maier 1967)* – When an event occurs independen your actions, it can be the basic cause of learned helplessness. Three causal attributions: 1) inte vs. external – personal internal factors vs. external fate or bad luck; 2) global vs. specific —attr failure to wide range of situations vs. being unsuccessful with specific factor; 3) stable vs unsta learned helplessness occurring occasionally or consistently over time. Suggests that interventic needs to emphasize cognitive and emotional as well as behavioral ways of handling uncertainty

Persuasion in Communications *(McGuire)* – Individuals pass through a series of ste order to assimilate a desired behavior: Exposure to the message; attention to message; interest in or personal relevance of message; understanding; personalizing behavior to fit life; accepting change; remembering the message and continuing to agree with it; being able to think of it; making decisions based on bringing the message to mind; behaving as decided; receiving (positive) reinforcement for behavior; accepting the behavior into one's life.

To communicate the message successfully, five communication components all must work: the credibility of the message source; the message design; the delivery channel; the target audience; the targeted behavior.

SMCR THEORY *(Berlo 1960)* –

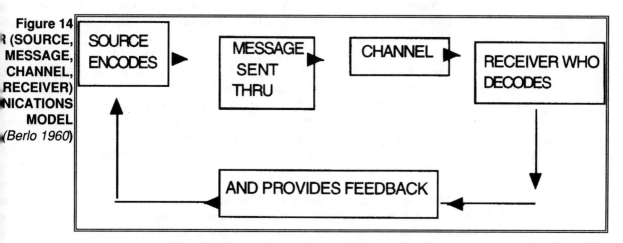

Figure 14
SMCR (SOURCE, MESSAGE, CHANNEL, RECEIVER) COMMUNICATIONS MODEL *(Berlo 1960)*

CHARACTERISTICS OF SOURCE- credibility, likeability, similarity
CHARACTERISTICS OF MESSAGE- order (first or last); one-side or 2; fear; visuals; amount of evidence, etc.
CHARACTERISTICS OF CHANNEL- one medium vs. other, combinations, keep message simple, noise or distraction
CHARACTERISTICS OF RECEIVER- personality variables (self-esteem efficacy, anxiety, ego-defensiveness) ego-involvement (emotional commitment)

PRECEDE *(Green, Kreuter, et al)* – A planning model with four steps: a social diagnosis, epidemiological diagnosis, behavioral and environmental diagnosis, and an educational and organizational diagnosis. In the educational and organizational diagnosis phase, predisposing, enabling, and reinforcing factors (from which the PRECEDE acronym is derived) a thorough behavior change analysis is carried out. In the 1991 edition of this book, a 5th step, policy, regulatory, and organizational analysis (PROCEED) has been added that provides the environmental, resources, and political diagnosis required for change.

Self-Efficacy Theory *(Bandura 1986)* – Perceived self-efficacy is defined as people's judgme[nt of] their capabilities to organize and execute courses of action required to attain designated types o[f] performance. It is concerned not with the skills one has but with judgments or beliefs of what o[ne can] do with whatever skills one possesses. It is behavior specific. You can have high efficacy for o[ne] behavior and low for another. Deals with our perception or belief that we can accomplish some behavior—in this way it is predictive.

We can change self-efficacy: by skills mastery – good way to accomplish mastery is to [have] clients contract for specific behaviors, and give feedback; modelling – see someone else perform[ing] coping or let group members solve problems; reinterpretation of physiological signs and sympt[oms] – identify beliefs and reinterpret them; persuasion – urge toward short-term realistic goals and en[list] high credibility persuaders.

Social Learning Theory *(Bandura)* – (a.k.a. Social Cognitive Theory) Sharp contras[t to] behaviorism and is integrative, focusing on cognitive theories which emphasize internal factors [such] as attitudes, values, beliefs (we learn how to behave from our social interactions) and external determinants of behavior. Major concepts include: environment, situation (person's perception[)], behavioral capability, expectation, expectancies, self-control, observational learning, reinforce[ment,] self-efficacy, emotional coping responses, reciprocal determinism (the dynamic interaction of p[erson,] behavior, and environment).

Stages of Change *(Prochaska & DiClemente)* – assumption that chronic behavior do[es not] change all at once, but on a continuum: 1) precontemplation – no interest, not thinking about ch[ange]; 2) contemplation – serious thought given to change; 3) action – 6 month period after overt actio[n is] taken; 4) maintenance – from 6 months to whenever behavioral problem is terminated (either b[y] habit or relapse).

104

THE HEALTH EDUCATION SP[

SELF-ASSESSMENT FOR HEALTH EDUCATORS

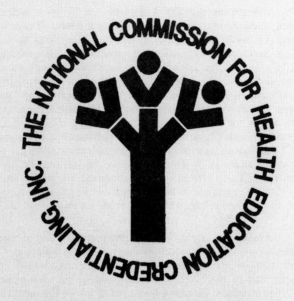

NATIONAL COMMISSION
FOR
HEALTH EDUCATION CREDENTIALING, INC.

Offices located at:

Professional Examination Service
Room 740
475 Riverside Drive
New York, NY 10115

There is general agreement that health education must play a large role if the nation is to meet its health objectives for the year 2000. There probably has been no greater opportunity than the present for health educators to demonstrate their worth. To be effective they must be able to assume a number of responsibilities with competency and skill. The instruments in this document can be very helpful aids to that end.

When using the *Self Assessment for Health Educators - Perceived Competence* instrument, the individual is asked to indicate the level of competence one feels in a particular skill area. The skills addressed represent those identified by the National Commission for Health Education Credentialing, Inc. as essential for the generic, entry level health educator (i.e. skills necessary for any entry level health educator to have no matter what the work setting). The skills emanate from the seven areas of responsibility and their related competencies which appear in *A Framework for the Development of Competency-based Curricula for Entry Level Health Educators*. The areas of responsibility are: 1) Assessing individual and community needs for health education; 2) Planning effective health education programs; 3) Implementing health education programs; 4) Evaluating effectiveness of health education programs; 5) Coordinating provision of health education services; 6) Acting as a resource person in health education; 7) Communicating health and health education needs, concerns, and resources. These responsibilities, competencies, and skills resulted from careful deliberation by virtually hundreds of health educators and health care providers in a role delineation, role verification and refinement, and curriculum framework development process.

Among the several uses for this particular self assessment instrument are the following: 1) A professional preparation program might administer it to their graduating students to determine where the strengths and weaknesses in their curriculum lie. Accordingly, adjustments can be made. 2) Individuals can use the instrument as a mechanism for determining what professional literature they need to spend the most time with in preparing for taking the National Commission for Health Education Credentialing, Inc. certification examination. 3) Employers and professional health education organizations will find the instrument useful when establishing priorities for continuing education offerings.

The second instrument in this document is entitled, *Self Assessment for Health Educators - Practical Application*. In this case the health educator is asked to indicate how useful each competency is perceived to be in that individual's current area of responsibility. It is conceivable that in a particular work situation a health educator may not need to be competent in all the seven areas of responsibility delineated as necessary for the generic health educator. It would be valuable for that individual to know the areas that are not deemed important -- or that are outside of his/her realm of responsibility. This individual may be able to demonstrate to an employer that the health educator in this agency could assume greater responsibility. This same individual could determine what areas in which competency must be maintained in planning to move into another health education position. Likewise, feedback from individuals who use this instrument can help the National Commission in its periodic revision of its curriculum framework. It is assumed that over time areas of responsibility as well as competencies and their related skills will need to be altered as society, the work setting, and technology change.

Individuals and groups will find additional purposes for using these instruments. If health educators are to be valued professionals in our society, it is essential that they regularly examine the effectiveness of their activities. This document provides an opportunity to do just that.

SELF ASSESSMENT FOR HEALTH EDUCATORS

Perceived Competence

The competency statements you are asked to respond to in this assessment describe the broadly defined skills that a qualified entry-level, generic health educator is expected to be able to demonstrate at least at minimum levels.

To assess your individual skill level for each competency statement you are asked to rate each competency from 1 to 4, with 1 indicating you do not feel competent in that skill area to 4 that you feel very competent in that skill.

| not | very |
| competent | competent |

1   2   3   4

SELF ASSESSMENT FOR HEALTH EDUCATORS

RESPONSIBILITY I: The health educator, working with individuals, groups, and organization responsible for:

Assessing individual and community needs for health education.

The health educator can:

Competency A: Obtain health related data about social and cultural environments, growth and development factors, needs, and interests.

	not competent			very comp
1. Select valid sources of information about health needs and health knowledge.	1	2	3	4
2. Utilize computerized sources of health-related information.	1	2	3	4
3. Employ or develop appropriate data-gathering information.	1	2	3	4
4. Apply survey techniques to acquire health data.	1	2	3	4

Competency B: Distinguish between behaviors that foster and those that hinder well-being.

1. Investigate physical, social, emotional, and intellectual factors influencing health behaviors.	1	2	3	4
2. Identify behaviors that tend to promote or compromise health.	1	2	3	4
3. Recognize the role of learning and affective experiences in shaping patterns of health behavior.	1	2	3	4

Competency C: Infer needs for health education on the basis of obtained data.

1. Examine needs assessment data.	1	2	3	4
2. Determine priority areas of need for health education.	1	2	3	4

RESPONSIBILITY II: The health educator, working with individuals, groups, and organizations is responsible for:

Planning effective health education programs.

The health educator can:

Competency A: Recruit community organizations, resource people, and potential participants for support and assistance in program planning.

	not competent		very competent	
1. Communicate need for the program to those whose cooperation will be essential.	1	2	3	4
2. Obtain commitments from personnel and decision makers who will be involved in the program.	1	2	3	4
3. Seek ideas and opinions of those who will affect or be affected by the program.	1	2	3	4
4. Incorporate feasible ideas and recommendations into the planning process.	1	2	3	4

Competency B: Develop a logical scope and sequence plan for a health education program.

1. Determine the range of health information requisite to a given program of instruction.	1	2	3	4
2. Organize the subject areas comprising the scope of a program in logical sequence.	1	2	3	4

Competency C: Formulate appropriate and measurable program objectives.

1. Infer educational objectives facilitative of achievement of specified competencies.	1	2	3	4
2. Develop a framework of broadly stated, operational objectives relevant to a proposed health education program.	1	2	3	4

Competency D: Design educational programs consistent with specified program objectives.

1. Match proposed learning activities with those implicit in the stated objectives.	1	2	3	4
2. Formulate a wide variety of alternative educational methods.	1	2	3	4
3. Select strategies best suited to implementation of educational objectives in a given setting.	1	2	3	4
4. Plan a sequence of learning opportunities building upon and reinforcing mastery of preceding objectives.	1	2	3	4

RESPONSIBILITY III: The health educator, working with individuals, groups, and organiz:
is responsible for:
Implementing health education programs.

The health educator can:
Competency A: Exhibit competence in carrying out planned educational programs.

	not competent		very comp	
1. Employ a wide range of educational methods and techniques.	1	2	3	4
2. Apply individual or group process methods as appropriate to given learning situations.	1	2	3	4
3. Utilize instructional equipment and other instructional media effectively.	1	2	3	4
4. Select methods that best facilitate practice of program objectives.	1	2	3	4

Competency B: Infer enabling objectives as needed to implement instructional programs in specified settings.

1. Pretest learners to ascertain present abilities and knowledge relative to proposed program objectives.	1	2	3	4
2. Develop subordinate measurable objectives as needed for instruction.	1	2	3	4

Competency C: Select methods and media best suited to implement program plans for specific learners.

1. Analyze learner characteristics, legal aspects, feasibility, and other considerations influencing choices among methods.	1	2	3	4
2. Evaluate the efficacy of alternative methods and techniques capable of facilitating program objectives.	1	2	3	4
3. Determine the availability of information, personnel, time, and equipment needed to implement the program for a given audience.	1	2	3	4

Competency D: Monitor educational programs, adjusting objectives and activities as necessary.

1. Compare actual program activities with the state objectives.	1	2	3	4
2. Assess the relevance of existing program objectives to current needs.	1	2	3	4
3. Revise program activities and objectives as necessitated by changes in learner needs.	1	2	3	4
4. Appraise applicability of resources and materials relative to given educational objectives.	1	2	3	4

RESPONSIBILITY IV: The health educator, working with individuals, groups, and organizations is responsible for:
Evaluating effectiveness of health education program.

The health educator can:
Competency A: Develop plans to assess achievement of program objectives.

	not competent		very competent	
1. Determine standards of performance to be applied as criteria of effectiveness.	1	2	3	4
2. Establish a realistic scope of evaluation efforts.	1	2	3	4
3. Develop an inventory of existing valid and reliable tests and survey instruments.	1	2	3	4
4. Select appropriate methods for evaluating program effectiveness.	1	2	3	4

Competency B: Carry out evaluation plans.

1. Facilitate administration of the tests and activities specified in the plan.	1	2	3	4
2. Utilize data collecting methods appropriate to the objectives.	1	2	3	4
3. Analyze resulting evaluation data.	1	2	3	4

Competency C: Interpret results of program evaluation.

1. Apply criteria of effectiveness to obtained results of a program.	1	2	3	4
2. Translate evaluation results into terms easily understood by others.	1	2	3	4
3. Report effectiveness of educational programs in achieving proposed objectives.	1	2	3	4

Competency D: Infer implications from findings for future program planning.

1. Explore possible explanations for important evaluation findings.	1	2	3	4
2. Recommend strategies for implementing results of evaluation.	1	2	3	4

RESPONSIBILITY V: The health educator working with individuals, groups, and organiza
is responsible for:
  Coordinating provisions of health education services.

  The health educator can:
    Competency A: Develop a plan for coordinating health education services.

	not competent			v com
1. Determine the extent of available health education services.	1	2	3	4
2. Match health education services to proposed program activities.	1	2	3	4
3. Identify gaps and overlaps in the provision of collaborative health services.	1	2	3	4

    Competency B: Facilitate cooperation between and among levels
                  of program personnel.

1. Promote cooperation and feedback among personnel related to the program.	1	2	3	4
2. Apply various methods of conflict reduction as needed.	1	2	3	4
3. Analyze the role of health educator as liaison between program staff and outside groups and organizations.	1	2	3	4

    Competency C: Formulate practical modes of collaboration among
                  the health agencies and organizations.

1. Stimulate development of cooperation among personnel responsible for community health education programs.	1	2	3	4
2. Suggest approaches for integrating health education within existing health programs.	1	2	3	4
3. Develop plans for promoting collaborative efforts among health agencies and organizations with mutual interests.	1	2	3	4

    Competency D: Organize inservice training programs for teachers,
                  volunteers, and other interested personnel.

1. Plan an operational, competency oriented training program.	1	2	3	4
2. Utilize instructional resources that meet a variety of inservice training needs.	1	2	3	4
3. Demonstrate a wide range of strategies for conducting inservice training programs.	1	2	3	4

RESPONSIBILITY VI: The health educator, working with individuals, groups and organizations is responsible for:
   Acting as a resource person in health education.

   The health educator can:
   Competency A: Utilize computerized health information retrieval systems effectively.

	not competent		very competent	
1. Match an information need with the appropriate retrieval system.	1	2	3	4
2. Access principal online and other databased health information resources.	1	2	3	4

   Competency B: Establish effective consultative relationships with those requesting assistance in solving health-related problems.

1. Analyze parameters of effective consultative relationships.	1	2	3	4
2. Describe special skills and abilities needed by health educators for consultation activities.	1	2	3	4
3. Formulate a plan for providing consultation to other health professionals.	1	2	3	4
4. Explain the process of marketing health education consultative services.	1	2	3	4

   Competency C: Interpret and respond to requests for health information.

1. Analyze general processes for identifying the information needed to satisfy a request.	1	2	3	4
2. Employ a wide range of approaches in referring requesters to valid sources of health information.	1	2	3	4

   Competency D: Select effective educational resource materials for dissemination.

1. Assemble educational material of value to the health of individuals and community groups.	1	2	3	4
2. Evaluate the worth and applicability of resource materials for given audiences.	1	2	3	4
3. Apply various processes in the acquisition of resource materials.	1	2	3	4
4. Compare different methods for distributing educational materials.	1	2	3	4

RESPONSIBILITY VII: The health educator, working with individuals, groups, and organizations is responsible for:

Communicating health and health education needs, concerns, and resources.

The health educator can:

Competency A: Interpret concepts, purposes, and theories of health education.

	not competent			v competent
1. Evaluate the state of the art of health education.	1	2	3	4
2. Analyze the foundations of the discipline of health education.	1	2	3	4
3. Describe major responsibilities of the health education in the practice of health education.	1	2	3	4

Competency B: Predict the impact of societal value systems on health education programs.

1. Investigate social forces causing opposing viewpoints regarding health education needs and concerns.	1	2	3	4
2. Employ a wide range of strategies for dealing with controversial health issues.	1	2	3	4

Competency C: Select a variety of communication methods and techniques in providing health information.

1. Utilize a wide range of techniques for communicating health and health education information and education.	1	2	3	4
2. Demonstrate proficiency in communicating health information and health education needs.	1	2	3	4

Competency D: Foster communication between health care providers and consumers.

1. Identify the significance and implications of health care providers' messages to consumers.	1	2	3	4
2. Act as liaison between consumer groups and individuals, and health care provider organizations.	1	2	3	4

INFORMATION ON C.H.E.S. & N.C.H.E.C.

Certified Health Education Specialist (C.H.E.S.)

Certification grants recognition to an individual who has met the qualifications for the entry-level health education professional. The standards have been specified by seven professional health education organizations and individual health educators. Further information on the standards is available in "A Framework for the Development of Competency-based Curricula for Entry-level Health Educators," available through NCHEC.

Delineating the scope of practice has benefits for the profession, the employer, and for the individual health educator.

Those eligible for the examination must have a degree from an accredited institution of higher education with a health education emphasis (minimum of 25 semester hour credits or 37 quarter hour credits). All seven areas of responsibility for the entry-level health educator that are listed in this text are to be included in the training.

The Commission has three purposes: 1) to certify health education specialists; 2) to promote professional development; and 3) to strengthen professional preparation.

For additional information on the examination or on the Commission's other activities, contact the Commission at the address below.

THE NATIONAL COMMISSION
FOR HEALTH EDUCATION CREDENTIALING, INC.
PROFESSIONAL EXAMINATION SERVICE
475 RIVERSIDE DRIVE, SUITE 740
NEW YORK, NEW YORK 10115
TEL - (212) 870-2047

SHORT READING LIST FOR THE HEALTH EDUCATION EXAM

Breckon, D., J. Harvey, and R. B. Lancaster. <u>Community Health Education: Settings, Roles, & Skills.</u> 2nd ed. Rockville, Md.: Aspen Systems, 1989. Health educator roles, skills, and settings addressed to the health education competencies.

Craig, D.P. <u>Hip Pocket Guide to Planning and Evaluation.</u> San Diego: University Associates, 1978.

Fodor, J.T., and G. T. Dalis. <u>Health Instruction: Theory and Application.</u> 4th ed. Philadelphia: Lea & Febiger, 1989.

Glanz, K., F.M. Lewis, and B. K. Rimer. <u>Health Behavior and Health Education: Theory, Research, and Practice.</u> San Francisco: Jossey-Bass, 1990.

Green, L.W., and M.W. Kreuter. <u>Health Promotion Planning: An Educational and Environmental Approach.</u> 2nd ed. Palo Alto, Ca.: Mayfield, 1991. Expands PRECEDE model to more comprehensive field of health promotion, adding PROCEED (policy, regulatory, & organizational constructs). Good site specific applications.

Green, L.W., M.W. Kreuter, S.G. Deeds, and K.B. Partridge. <u>Health Education Planning: A Diagnostic Approach.</u> Palo Alto, Ca.: Mayfield, 1980. Presents the PRECEDE framework as an organizing framework to sort out the complexities of planning health education programs.

Greene, W.H., and B.G. Simons-Morton. <u>Introduction to Health Education.</u> Prospect Heights, Ill.: Waveland Press, 1990. Throrough introduction to the subject of health education. Recommended as best overall introduction.

<u>Healthy People 2000: National Health Promotion and Disease Prevention Objectives.</u> U.S. DHHS, PHS 1990 DHHS Pub # (PHS) 91-505212. Washington, D.C.: U.S. GPO, 1990.

Pickett, G., and J. Hanlon. <u>Public Health: Administration and Practice.</u> St. Louis, Mo.: Times Mirror/Mosby, 1990.

The fastest way to buy a book if you can't find it in the library or a college bookstore is to call information (1-800-555-1212) to get the publisher's toll-free number. Call the order desk and use your credit card.

ABOUT THE AUTHOR

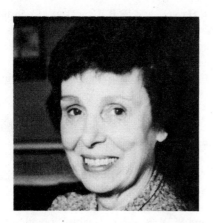

Sigrid G. Deeds Dr.P.H., C.H.E.S., developed
tested this manual based on her twentysome years of health educatio
practice. She has been an author, consultant, and teacher and has
practiced in state and county health departments, voluntary agencies,
medical care and corporate settings. She served as national Presiden
the Society for Public Health Education, Editor of Health Education
Monographs (now HEQ), Chair of the Public Health Education and
Health Promotion Section, and on the Governing Council of the
American Public Health Association.

Dr. Deeds is currently Professor of Community Health at California
University, Long Beach, California.